Reframing Contemporary Physician Leadership

We Started as Heroes

Grace E. Terrell, MD, MMM,
CPE, FACP, FACPE

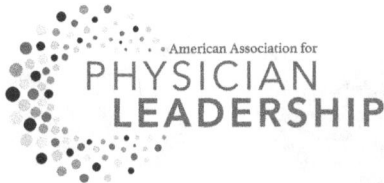

American Association for
PHYSICIAN
LEADERSHIP

AAPL books are available at special quantity discounts to use as premiums and sales
promotions, or for use in corporate training programs. For more information, please
write to Special Sales at journal@physicianleaders.org

This publication is designed to provide general information and is sold with the
understanding that neither the author nor the publisher is engaged in rendering legal,
accounting, ethical, or clinical advice. If legal or other expert advice is required, the
services of a competent professional person should be sought.

13   8 7 6 5 4 3 2 1

Copyedited, typeset, indexed, and printed in the United States of America

PUBLISHER
Nancy Collins

EDITORIAL ASSISTANT
Jennifer Weiss

DESIGN & LAYOUT
Carter Publishing Studio

COPYEDITOR
Pat George

To Gabriella Emily Garrison, with love.

ACKNOWLEDGMENTS

I am so grateful to the 11 outstanding physician leaders who shared their personal stories with me and have allowed me to tell you about them. In all of their interviews, these leaders were authentic, humble, and openly vulnerable. I have been inspired by each of them during my medical career and believe you will be, too.

Thank you very much, David Bick, MD; Jennifer Byrne, MD, PhD; Dekarlos Dial, DPM; Jesse James, MD, MBA; Alan Kaplan, MD, MMM, FACPE, FACHE; Eugenie Komives, MD; Kavita Patel, MD, MSHS; Jerry Penso, MD, MBA; Scott Ransom, DO, MPH, MBA; Elisabeth Stambaugh, MD, MMM; and Elliott Williams, MD.

Throughout the long process of making the initial idea into a book, I have relied on the expert guidance of my publisher, Nancy Collins, and her excellent team of Jennifer Weiss and Patricia George at the American Association for Physician Leadership. Once again, they have been a delight to work with.

AAPL has been part of my life since 1995, when I joined what was then called the American College of Physician Executives and signed up for the Physicians in Management courses, parts 1, 2, and 3, as I began my personal physician leadership journey. I have learned so much from the many colleagues from around the country in meetings and classes at AAPL, and enthusiastically continue to encourage my physician colleagues to utilize AAPL's excellent resources. www.physicianleaders.org

I remain so thankful to J.M. Bohn, who co-authored with me *MD 2.0: Physician Leadership for the Information Age* in 2012 in my first exploration of physician leadership. Their non-physician perspective broadened my views and enriched our message.

I am indebted to all the leaders on the various leadership teams I have been part of through the years, including AAPL, AMGA, CCHIT, CHESS, Cornerstone Health Care, Envision Genomics, Eventus Whole Health, High Point Regional Health System, IKS Health, Kailos Genetics, NC Shakespeare Festival, PTAC, the Oliver Wyman Healthcare Leadership Alliance, and the High Point United Way. I have learned so much from "all y'all" as we say here in the South.

Finally, I am grateful to my original medical partners and in-laws, Drs. Eugene and Eldora Terrell, who taught me physician leadership lessons like the rock stars they are, my husband Tim, my parents and siblings, sons-in-laws and daughters, and now, best of all, baby Gabriella, who continue to inspire me to make my work about designing a better healthcare delivery system for now and for tomorrow.

TABLE OF CONTENTS

PART II: THE FUTURE IS OURS TO MAKE

PART III: LEADERSHIP PROFILES IN ACTION

ABOUT THE AUTHOR

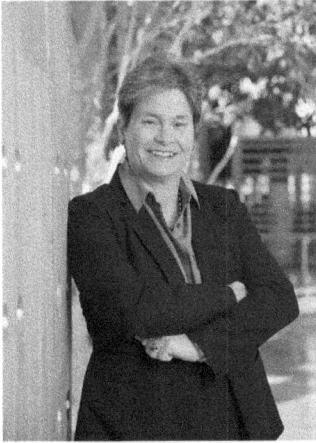

Grace E. Terrell, MD, MMM, CPE, FACP, FACPE, is a national thought leader in healthcare innovation and delivery system reform, and a serial entrepreneur in population health outcomes driven through patient care model design, clinical and information integration, and value-based payment models. She is also a practicing general internist.

She has served as CEO of Eventus WholeHealth, LLC, a company focused on providing holistic care to medically vulnerable adults. She is the former CEO of Cornerstone Health Care, one of the first medical groups to make the "move to value" by lowering the cost of care and improving its quality for the sickest, most vulnerable patients; the founding CEO of CHESS, a population health management company; and the former CEO of Envision Genomics, a company focused on the integration of precision medicine technology into population health frameworks for patients with rare and undiagnosed diseases.

Dr. Terrell has served as vice chair of the U.S. DHHS' Physician-Focused Payment Model Technical Advisory Committee, the chairman of the board of the AMGA, is a founding member of the Oliver Wyman Health Innovation Center, and the co-author of *Value-Based Care and Payment Models*.

She currently is executive in residence at Duke University School of Medicine's Master in Management of Clinical Informatics Program and a senior advisor for Oliver Wyman management consulting firm.

Physician Identities and Leadership Roles

About 10 years ago, I sat down to write a book that explored how the current environment was changing physicians, with the goal of providing some insight into the leadership challenges inculcated by the pace of the health delivery system transformation. I was worried that the traditional training physicians endured and the traditional social roles physicians occupied inadequately prepared us to be the leaders our nation's healthcare delivery system required for better performance.

Amid the acceleration of healthcare payment reform, rapid technologic change, and cultural challenges to the traditional sources of physician power, physician leaders needed new skills and behaviors. I believed that understanding physicians' historical and contemporary social identities within our culture was crucial to solving the leadership predicament physicians faced. So, I set about to explore and write about these issues.

My co-author, J.M. Bohn, and I wrote *MD 2.0: Physician Leadership for the Information Age.* Looking back, I believe we were right in being concerned about the changes that physician leaders would face, but in my wildest dreams, I did not imagine the degree of those changes. Ten years later, we have seen industry consolidation accelerate, payment reform stall, social media engender anti-science narratives denying basic medical facts, and, of course, a global pandemic creating the greatest public health emergency of our lifetimes.

Interestingly, the term "hero" has resurfaced as the dominant metaphor in the public narrative of frontline medical workers treating patients with COVID-19. No longer a designation reserved just for physicians; the medical hero now includes all of our medical team members who face the hard day-to-day work of providing healthcare during the healthcare crisis. The social memes of tired doctors and nurses in masks and scrubs are ubiquitous.

In *MD 2.0*, I deliberately challenged the physician-as-hero metaphor as being inadequate for the leadership skills required for what lay before us. The traditional role of healer has certain shamanistic characteristics that "hero" does not capture. And heroes are not always the archetype of leadership we need. I still believe that.

I introduced the Cherokee term "**duyukdv**" in the book to push for a broader understanding of physician identities and leadership roles. In the past ten years there has been increasing attention paid to the cultural appropriation of words ands symbols by dominant Western society from other cultures in ways that inappropriately co-opt their meaning for new or different purposes. I am not ethnically Cherokee. I simply believe that this word more holisticly engenders the qualities that I believe contemporary medical professionalism must embrace. As I understand it, **duyukdv** is the concept of "*living one's life in the right way and balancing the rights of the individual with the good of the whole.*" That concept is far broader than the concept of hero and, from my perspective, elaborates the form that physician professionalism and leadership need to take as we face the ongoing metamorphosis of what it means to be a physician in 21st century America.

Built upon the work I did 10 years ago and informed by 10 more years of experience in the trenches of the healthcare delivery system, this book re-explores some of the same themes from *MD 2.0*, albeit from a perspective more focused on the different identities physicians take on professionally and the ways they can be leaders within those various identities. As in the previous effort, I provide vignettes of real-life physicians who have embodied various forms of physician leadership.

In my own thinking, even the term "physician" needs to be expanded, not simply to include allopathic and osteopathic physicians, but also other clinician leaders who now comprise the medical profession. The Merriam-Webster definition of physician is "*a person skilled in the art of healing, specifically, one educated, clinically, experienced, and licensed to practice medicine. . . .*" Defensibly, that definition should include nurse practitioners, physician assistants/associates, podiatrists, and other healthcare providers with a scope of practice encompassed in the term "medicine." However, the recent hullabaloo wrought by physician assistants changing the name of their profession to physician associates and the ongoing controversy surrounding the use of the term "doctor" by nurse practitioners who have earned a doctorate demonstrates that ongoing authority, status, and scope of practice controversies remain.

Much of the analysis in this book is still deliberately focused on the more traditional understanding of physicians as being those who are doctors of medicine (either allopathic or osteopathic medicine), because understanding the particular social and cultural history of the profession is crucial in identifying the barriers to and opportunities for the needed good leadership often lamented as diminished within the traditional physician role.

The scope and scale of leadership that our healthcare delivery system craves, nonetheless, requires a far larger team than the just over 1 million individuals in the United States with an active medical license who make up our physician workforce. I hope the re-exploration of the themes of physician leadership within this broader context will be useful for all of our clinicians in preparing for and participating in the crucial professional functions needed to fulfill the expansive oath to *"first do no harm."*

The more accurate translation of the Hippocratic oath is to *"do no harm or injustice to them."*[1] From my perspective, this admonishment is a calling more than an oath, and its fulfillment is more expansive than traditional bedside care of the sick. Imbedded in the professional roles we take on as physicians is the duty to avoid *injustice* in the rendering of our services. That duty is rarely acknowledged explicitly if it is understood at all. If we are to move forward with an improved model of physician professionalism, it must be.

I hope this book will help in the effort to reframe physician professionalism within a broader scope that includes the avoidance of injustice by yoking professionalism directly to leadership, and by illuminating both the barriers and pathways to new professionalism built upon leadership.

---

1. National Library of Medicine. Greek Medicine. National Library of Medicine-National Institutes of Health. www.nlm.nih.gov/hmd/greek/greek_oath.html. Retrieved 10 January 2021.

PART I

Condition Red: Situation Today

CHAPTER 1

Where We Stand

The dogmas of the quiet past are inadequate to the stormy present. The occasion is piled high with difficulty. As our case is new, so we must think anew and act anew. We must disenthrall ourselves, and then we shall save our country.[1]

President Abraham Lincoln
1862 Address to Congress

So here we are. Two years after the first reported cases of SARS-CoV-2 in the United States, more than 813,000 Americans have died, 57.7 million have been confirmed with the illness, and we have experienced the greatest decline in the economy since the Great Depression. The U.S. healthcare delivery system has reeled under the pressures of the pandemic, from the initial inadequate testing and personal protective equipment capabilities to layoffs resulting from the postponement of elective procedures and inadequate cash flow built upon fee-for-service revenues.

Even as ICUs overflow with COVID-19 patients requiring ventilatory support, death rates in patients without a COVID diagnosis have substantially increased, as people avoid or no longer have access to care for stroke, heart disease, cancer, and the other common serious medical illnesses. Many independent physician groups that were unable to sustain their business during the pandemic have been acquired by larger entities.

The horrifying death rates in long-term care facilities early in the pandemic led to lock-downs with their own horrific consequences, including residents' extreme depression and loneliness due to isolation from family and the wider community (Figure 1).

With the economy in shambles, many employees who depended on employer-sponsored health insurance lost access to healthcare along with their jobs. Children were not in school. Restaurants, sporting events, concerts, and theaters closed, and the airline industry is near bankruptcy. The nation has not experienced this degree of political upheaval since the Civil War.

After years of decline, U.S. death rate shot up in 2020

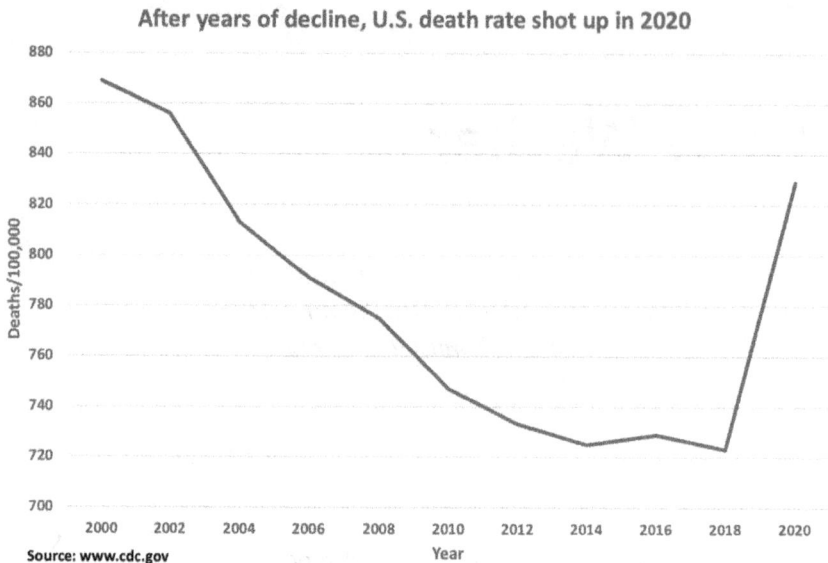

Figure 1. U.S. Death Rate 2000–2020. Source: The Centers for Disease Control and Prevention

Amid the existential professional crisis wrought by the COVID-19 pandemic, physician leadership has been on public display as never before. Dr. Anthony Fauci became an icon as the voice of medical authority in the Trump administration's White House Coronavirus Task Force and now as Chief Medical Advisor to President Joe Biden.[2]

The astonishingly rapid development of highly effective vaccines by U.S. drugmaker Pfizer with their German partner BioNTech highlighted the scientific work of a husband-wife physician team unseen since the early 20th-century work by Pierre and Marie Curie. As voices of authority from their national platforms, Dr. Robert Redfield of the CDC, Dr. Deborah Birx of the White House Coronavirus Task Force, and Dr. Scott Atlas of Fox News and the White House Coronavirus Task Force have faced public adulation and condemnation. The pandemic led to the projection of physicians in the public eye as "heroes"[3] and unprecedented threats to public health officials who provided basic information to the public around pandemic safety practices.[4] Physicians around the world have been villainized and threatened by some members of the public.[5]

Physicians' identification as heroes has not rung true for many clinicians.[6] Even for the decades before the pandemic, physician burnout has been an increasing area of concern, with the physician persona of "superhero" identified as one of the factors leading to increasing levels of burnout.[7] Four hundred physicians die by suicide each year — double that of the general population; physicians have the highest rate of suicide of any profession in the United States.[8]

As Hartzband and Groopman have so aptly decried, "The unintended consequences of radical alterations in the healthcare system that were supposed to make physicians more efficient and productive, and thus more satisfied, have made them profoundly alienated and disillusioned."[9] These unintended consequences include electronic health records designed for billing rather than clinical ease of use, meaningless check-the-box performance measures, monetary penalties for expanding the length of face-to-face patient time, and reductions in professional authority and autonomy embedded in contemporary health system organizational structures and culture.

Despite the remarkable evidence of healthcare delivery system failure illuminated by the COVID-19 pandemic, the United States continues to spend a disproportionately high amount of money in the healthcare sector relative to other crucial components of our economy.

In 1960, U.S. federal government spending for education as a percentage of gross domestic product (GDP) was 3.7%; for defense, it was 10.1%; and for healthcare, it was 0.3%. By 2020, federal government spending as a percentage of GDP increased to 5.91% for education; defense spending decreased to 3.5%; and healthcare spending increased to 8.0%.[10] However, as a percentage of the overall federal budget, healthcare spending ballooned to 28% and is expected to accelerate to one-third of federal spending within the next eight years.[11] [12]

This degree of spending strains the capacity to invest in important aspects of government spending, including infrastructure, defense, education, and crucial challenges like climate change. The amount of money spent in the U.S. on healthcare privately is accelerating even more rapidly than governmental spending. Since 1960, the federal, state, and private expenditures for healthcare services and goods in the U.S. accelerated from 5.2% in 1960 to 18.0% in 2020 (Figure 2).

The passage of the Affordable Care Act in 2009 significantly reduced the percentage of uninsured Americans. While the uninsured segment of the American population stood at 49.7 million in 2010, the projected impact of insurance market reform that was forecast to bring this number down to 24.4 million by 2019 began to unravel with policy changes instituted during the Trump administration (Figure 3).[13]

US National Health Expenditures as % GDP

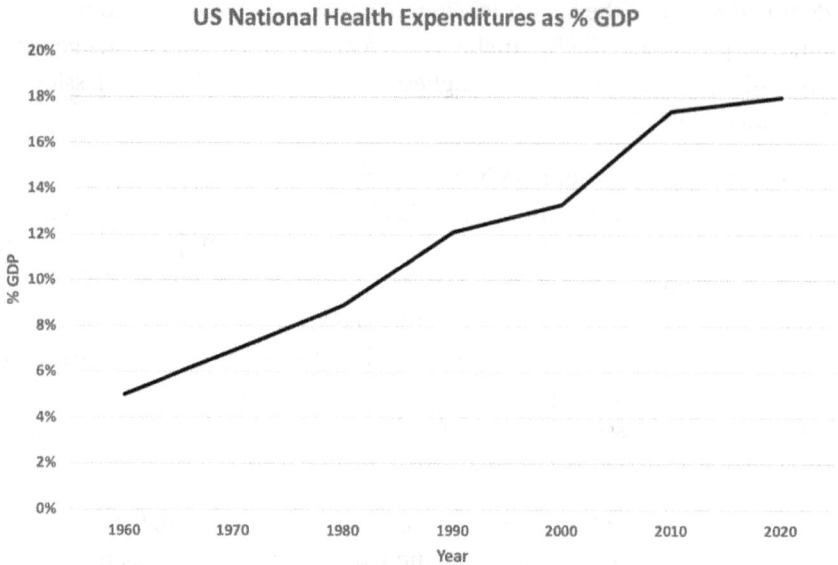

Figure 2. U.S. National Expenditures as Percentage of Gross Domestic Product, 1960–2020.

The uninsured population reached a nadir of 26.7 million Americans in 2016 (10.0% of the population) with gradual increases since,[14] substantially worsening during the pandemic due to loss of employer-sponsored insurance by the newly unemployed.[15] This uninsured population segment will continue to challenge healthcare providers when their lack of access to basic healthcare services inevitably leads them to the emergency departments of our overburdened hospitals or to reduced access to any healthcare at all.

More than two decades have passed since the release of the Institute of Medicine's (IOM) landmark report *To Err Is Human*[16] that spotlighted the high number of medical errors occurring throughout our health system. Even today, with significant resources having been dedicated by healthcare organizations, government agencies, not-for-profit organizations, and physician practices across the country to conduct major quality improvement initiatives, our nation's health system continues to face significant challenges with eliminating medical errors.

Medical errors remain a leading cause of death in the United States, costing $20 billion a year and resulting in 100,000 lives lost.[17] Prior to the pandemic, one study suggested medical errors may be the third-leading cause of death in the U.S. at 250,000 lives annually, surpassing respiratory diseases, which

**U.S. Nonelderly Uninsured Population
2010-2020**

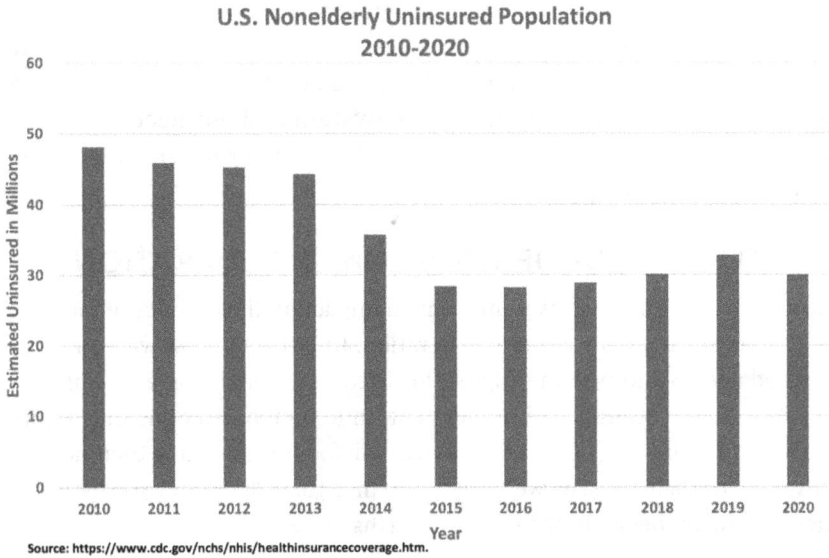

Source: https://www.cdc.gov/nchs/nhis/healthinsurancecoverage.htm.

Figure 3. U.S. Nonelderly Uninsured Population, 2010–2020. Source: Centers for Disease Control and Prevention National Center for Health Statistics

kill close to 150,000 people a year. Diagnostic errors, medical mistakes, and the absence of safety nets contribute to deaths that heretofore did not show up in national health statistics designed for billing coding.[18]

The inability to easily identify the consequences of medical errors in traditional healthcare statistics should not be surprising. Despite a decade-long push for delivery system reform built upon alternative payment models, the U.S. healthcare system largely remains a fee-for-service payment model. The economic incentives of a fee-for-service healthcare system drive overutilization of profitable services by healthcare providers, to which the private payers respond through managed care and the governmental payers respond through regulation.

These countermeasures to overutilization increasingly frustrate physicians and other healthcare providers, who perceive less freedom to practice medicine unfiltered by externally imposed constraints. Alongside the anxieties invoked by the current punitive tort-based malpractice system, physicians experience decreased professional morale due to the challenges of practicing in a highly managed and regulated environment. The current self-reported professional morale among physicians is dismal, with only 44.7% reporting "somewhat or very positive feeling about the current state of the medical profession."[19]

Regardless of professional morale, demographic and socioeconomic changes will continue to drive the healthcare delivery system reform, and it is imperative physicians prepare for and lead the changes to come. These changes serve as justification for continued innovation and our need for strong, diplomatic, and collaborative physician leaders to improve the health of our current and future population.

THE IMPACT OF THE BOOMER GENERATION

No generation will make as significant an impact on the practice of medicine in America as the baby boomer generation. In 2011, the first wave of babies reached age 65 and became eligible for Medicare benefits at a rate of 7,000 per day. As the 80 million boomers continue to age and consume greater portions of healthcare, American society will focus on meeting their needs at this stage of their lives, as we have done since their disproportionate demographic impact began in the post-war births in 1946.

During the 1950s and 1960s, when the boomers were younger, America focused on the "youth culture." Between the 1970s and the 2000s, the group focused on the socioeconomic issues of marriage, child-rearing, and work-life productivity. In 2011, the tides turned as the largest segment of American society began to grapple with the issues of retirement and aging.

We should not expect the baby boomers to "go gentle into that good night" any more than we should have expected them all to consent to the draft during the Vietnam War. This portion of the American population, with demographic strength in numbers, coupled with buying power and political strength, is reaching the point in their lifecycle when their increasing healthcare needs are becoming a top priority.

One could argue that the Clinton healthcare reform attempt of the early 1990s failed because the baby boomers were too young, healthy, and productive at that point in their lives for healthcare to rise to the top of federal political policy concerns.

Boomers were far more concerned in the 1990s with competing for good jobs and having a thriving economy than healthcare, as long as the cost of healthcare did not interfere with the more pressing economic demands of their early adulthood. During this decade, healthcare reforms that focused on cost-control ran up against employers competing for talent in the workforce with benefits focused on access and choice.

In the popular media, 1990s films like Robin William's *Patch Adams*, Danny DeVito's and Matt Damon's *The Rainmaker*, and Jack Nicholson's *As Good as*

It Gets derive part of their storyline from the tension between medical systems and health insurance companies limiting access to good healthcare. Employers competing for talent chose various forms of managed care to help control the costs of rich benefits plans and easy access the workforce demanded.

Now that they are aging, the baby boomer demographic inevitably will force healthcare policy reform, but as this population segment moves into its golden years, the 40 million generation X workers cannot replace the 80 million boomers in the workforce without radical structural changes or more liberal immigration policy. Although it became apparent decades ago that inefficiencies in the healthcare system would create a daunting challenge to meet the healthcare needs of aging boomers, it was not until they approached the years in which their Medicare entitlements kicked in that we began focusing on wellness and longevity research, changes in healthcare political agendas, renewed efforts in innovation across the gamut of care delivery, and modern technologies designed to keep the elderly independent.

Most importantly, the impending demographic wave of geriatric boomers will catalyze the transition away from the volume-driven care delivery system that emerged with the managed care era toward one that is more focused on the delivery of high-value and high-quality services. The economic boom and productivity gains in the U.S. economy in the 1990s correlated with the baby boomers' high-productivity work years. Employers were thus focused on competing for employees who offered rich benefits and managing the cost of doing so via managed care. Now those strategies are being applied in the Medicare Advantage market.

The healthcare delivery system needs physician leaders capable of rising to the occasion of the inevitable reforms in the industry wrought by the need to provide efficient healthcare services to 80 million older adults and younger Americans needing access to care, with lower life expectancies, greater cultural diversity, and fewer economic resources.

To do so, the physician profession itself will need to transform. The profession must face and solve the health consequences of climate change, racism, economic inequity, and chronic underfunding of our public health infrastructure. This complex macroenvironment requires our clinicians to have new, stronger leadership skills. To attain these skills, physicians must understand who they are within a broad historical context and develop the resilience, foresight, and creativity needed to lead in a fast-changing world that needs a far better healthcare delivery system than the one in which they currently practice.

AMERICA'S MEDICAL PROFESSION

The earliest archeological evidence reveals that humankind has always worked through cultural evolution to change the environment to meet our needs. Whether by developing rudimentary stone tools, transforming from hunter-gatherer to agricultural production, developing densely populated settlements, or advancing modern technology and scientific methodology, humankind has sought to improve our lives by changing our physical and social environment.

However, the consequences of our actions also led to unanticipated adverse environmental changes. With the advent of animal domestication and the rise of dense populations of relatively sedentary groups of people, rich niches for rodents, parasites, and insects developed, and disease patterns changed. New dependence on a grain-based diet subject to putrefaction in storage exposed humans to new bacteria, molds, and toxins. The more narrowed nutritional spectrum of the agriculturally derived grain-based diet also led to nutritional deficiencies in vitamins, proteins, and minerals, and in times of poor crop yield, starvation.

Whereas evidence of the treatment of trauma has been found in the earliest Paleolithic records, the advent of cities over the past 5,000 years has furthered the spread of epidemic infectious diseases derived from viruses, bacteria, and parasites. In the modern era, civilization exposes us to chemical and industrial toxins, radiation, alcohol and drug addiction, and an increase in the prevalence of other lifestyle-influenced diseases such as diabetes, cardiovascular disease, and cancer.

As long as human cultures have evolved and adapted to their physical and social environment, humankind has sought to maintain some control over disease. Anthropologists have identified the healer role across cultural boundaries as one way cultures attempt to understand, influence, and control human disease.

The earliest historical records of Egypt and Mesopotamia document an understanding of illness as a divine punishment for sins committed by the patient. The healer in cultures as diverse as those in native New World populations, Asia, Africa, Europe, and Oceania can be described as a shaman whose cultural purpose is to serve as a mediator with the spirit world to relieve the physical distress of a suffering individual. The shaman holds cultural power by bridging the natural world and the spiritual world to benefit the community.[20]

In modern Western culture, the scientific revolution led to a rationalist approach to physical disease and, as Paul Starr articulates in his introduction in his 1982 book *The Social Transformation of American Medicine:*

> Though the works of reason have lifted innumerable burdens of hunger and sorrow, they have also cast up a new world of power. In that world, some people stand above others in knowledge and authority and in control of the vast institutions that have arisen to manage and finance the rationalized forms of human labor.[21]

Starr's Pulitzer Prize-winning work analyzes the physician's role in American society from the colonial period until the advent of managed care in the 1980s. He describes physicians' rise in status based on their control and exploitation of emerging innovations in technologies and practices grounded in research, scientific evidence, and medical education. The resulting improvement in medical treatment accelerated the perceived value of the medical profession in America during the past 100 years.

Starr discusses the important role of medical education in the United States and the historical significance of the Flexner Report of 1910, which led to national physician curriculum standardization emphasizing the scientific method as critical to ethical high-quality patient care. The standardization of curricula emphasizing scientific inquiry helped improve the abilities of our nation's physicians to continually improve patient care through the development of evidence-based orders, guidelines, and practices.

Starr analyzes the complexities of how the physician profession rose to the level of power and authority in the United States that we see today. He argues that modern medicine has developed "an elaborate system of specialized knowledge, technical procedures, and rules of behavior," granting to the medical profession an especially persuasive claim to authority.

> Even among the sciences, medicine occupies a special position. Its practitioners come into direct and intimate contact with people in their daily lives; they are present at the critical transitional moments of existence. They serve as intermediaries between science and private experiences, interpreting personal troubles in the abstract language of scientific knowledge.[22]

Starr's analysis focuses on the sources of power in the medical profession leading to cultural authority and occupational control, economic power, and professional autonomy that was at its peak at the time of publication. He accurately predicted the current threats to professional sovereignty through "competition and control" as "hospitals and other organizations merge into larger and more powerful corporate systems . . . and beyond private bureaucratic organizations looms the regulatory power of the state and federal governments."[23]

Starr's analysis identifies the historical rise of power in the American medical profession and rightly points to the Flexner Report as a pivotal point in that rise. Others have emphasized the gender and racial consequences of the Flexner Report.

The Carnegie Foundation hired Abraham Flexner to conduct a survey to evaluate the quality of the 155 American medical schools operating in 1910. He recommended a reduction in the number of medical schools to 31, an increase in the prerequisites to enter medical training, training of physicians to practice via the scientific method, medical school control of clinical instruction in hospitals, and strengthened state regulation of medical licensure.

A major result of the post-Flexner reforms was the closing of all but two medical schools training African-American students, Howard University School of Medicine and Meharry Medical College.[24] The surviving medical schools did not quickly open their doors to women, African Americans, or other ethnic and religious minorities.[25] Consequentially, the medical profession increasingly became the dominion of white men, with the built-in social and financial elevated status of their entitlements.

Of course, Starr did not predict the impact of the Internet on patient access to information sources to help them make personal healthcare decisions without yielding to the authority of physicians and other healthcare service providers. Nor did his analysis foresee social media, where alternative narratives about the causes and cures of medical conditions compete directly with science-based authoritative sources of "truth."

Algorithms embedded in social media platforms influence the sources of information individuals seek. Along with the politicized algorithms of many social media platforms, the enormous power of search engines and artificial intelligence have accelerated the threats to professional authority embedded in the regulatory and economic management models.

Even with these limitations, Starr's analysis continues to be applicable in understanding the various economic and social factors physician leaders must address in critical decision-making for their own organizations and patient care decisions. The healthcare industry has been transformed organizationally through waves of vertical and horizontal integrations and mergers, with most physicians now employed by health systems or other large integrated delivery systems. However, even today, many physicians continue to operate as small business entrepreneurs, and alternative forms of practices, including telemedicine virtual models, home-based care models, and concierge medicine models, continue to be sources of innovation and practice diversity.

In the transitional state of contemporary medical practice, both the complex structures of large organizations and smaller entrepreneurial ventures are better understood within their historical context. Starr's analysis demonstrates the application of market dynamics in healthcare as a force for evolutional change within complex adaptive systems.

This implication that physicians have historically faced the market dynamics of their time permits a larger insight into the tension between the professional obligations of patient care and the economics of the community in which care is rendered.

Today, the market dynamics regulated through the Centers for Medicare and Medicaid Services, the Federal Trade Commission, the Food and Drug Administration, the Department of Justice, various state and local regulators, and commercial insurance constraints create an environment for medical practice in which physicians must adjust their objectives to improve access to care, affordability, and the quality of care, with the need to meet co-occurring interests of cooperation and competition as they occur within the financial market.[26]

The individual professional decisions made to achieve these objectives will involve economic impact issues (e.g., number of healthcare professionals to employ to meet consumer demand for services; impact of various supplier relations) and social relation issues (e.g., determining associations and advocacy agendas to support), some of which occur simultaneously and are collectively influenced by the actions taken by various stakeholders in our nation's healthcare community.

The "subtle loss of autonomy for the (medical) profession" resulting from the rise of corporations controlling the economics of the healthcare industry through "increasing corporate influence over the rules and standards of medical work" predicted by Starr in 1982 is old news now. He accurately foreshadowed that "the new generation of women physicians may find the new corporate organizations willing to allow more part-time and intermittent work than is possible in solo practice" and had the foresight to recognize that:

> There will be more regulation of the pace and routines of work. And the corporation is likely to require some standard of performance, whether measured in revenues generated or patients treated per hour.[27]

Starr did not predict the advent of the hospitalist movement, the rise of physician executives in a hybrid clinician/management role, or the regulation of resident physician work hours. However, these developments coincided with value-based healthcare that challenges the economic status quo in the healthcare delivery system.

The rise of managed care in the 1980s and 1990s that Starr describes is now evolving to include managed Medicare coincident with the aging population demographic changes and consumer-based healthcare delivery models that bypass traditional clinic- and hospital-based delivery models are rapidly gaining market share.

The tsunami of changes engendered by the Affordable Care Act (ACA), Health Information Technology for Economic and Clinical Health (HITECH) Act, the Medicare Access and CHIP Reauthorization Act (MACRA), and the 21st Century Cures Act coincide with the widespread consolidation of the industry through mergers and acquisitions, the development of patient-centered medical homes, and clinical integration among complementary provider organizations. Innovations in care delivery models naturally follow.

For the physicians and care providers in the medical profession, delivery system reform will accelerate organizational change and provide an opportunity to improve the continuity of care and result in a revitalized healthcare system going forward.

Alongside this potential renaissance, the information-system technology revolution offers us the opportunity for improvement in evidence-based medicine practices, communications, and stronger opportunities to deliver high-value care to patients. The necessity of keeping pace with continuous clinical advancement, new technologies, and increased reporting requirements will accelerate the rate of change in the healthcare delivery system. Physicians must both adapt and continue to provide the leadership and social authority to make these changes patient-centric or our special position in American healthcare will erode and become increasingly irrelevant.

THE PHYSICIAN'S COMPACT

The shamanistic healing role is a powerful one across many cultures. Still, the special authority physicians occupy in our culture is to a large extent dependent upon the long years of medical training where professional competencies develop that permit physicians to assert their professional authority within their own cultural context.

Physicians and other clinicians are exempted from social taboos within their professional roles related to physical contact and solicitation of confidential information from patients. Social aversions to disease, death, and decay are disregarded in order to restore health or relieve suffering. In doing so, physicians are allowed to probe the most intimate aspects of a patient's life for the purpose of healing or relieving pain to a far larger extent than other health-care workers have traditionally been permitted.

Within the confines of the professional relationship, physicians ask about a patient's bowel habits, sexual history, and the most private aspects of life. A surgeon opens the body to excise an infected appendix or breast malignancy within the proper clinical context of diagnosis and treatment without presumed boundary violation.

Stereotypically, contemporary Western physicians are recognized for their highly analytic academic achievement, diligence, perseverance, and self-abnegation. They are presumed to have the capacity for delayed gratification (i.e., status comes only after years of school and sacrifice), and the capacity to work without aversion when exposed to human suffering and disease.

A physician undergoes a prolonged apprenticeship; by the end of training, the physician is expected to effectively communicate with patients, be empathetic and discrete, and have flawless technical diagnostic and treatment skills. They will have been expected to work very long hours, sometimes neglecting food and sleep, sometimes delaying the adult roles of marriage and parenthood.

After four years of college, four years of medical school, a year-long internship, two to four years of medical residency, one to three years of fellowship for some specialists, and successful results on multiple licensing and competency exams, the long apprenticeship is completed. From a cultural perspective, this professional journey is a prolonged stage of adolescent development that is deemed necessary for professional expectations to be fulfilled.

Developmental psychologists delineate stages of life from infancy through adulthood that people must successfully navigate, one after another, in order to be prepared for the challenges of the next stages of life. Superimposed on these traditional developmental stages is the very long training journey of the medical profession. Physicians cannot successfully fill their ultimate professional roles and meet their challenges until they complete their prolonged training. Jean Piaget focused upon adolescence as a time of mastering concrete operations. Contemporary medical education requires mastering technical skills through many years of training, whether the skills are procedural, diagnostic, or therapeutic.

The professional identity of a physician as a fully licensed interventional cardiologist, for example, requires four years of college, four years of medical school, three years of an internal medicine residency, and four years of cardiology fellowship training. With no breaks in training, an 18-year-old high school graduate would be 33 years old before they had established an identity as an interventional cardiologist in the American medical education training system. In the traditional private practice model, the cardiologist subsequently has to complete the steps of passing boards and credentialing exams and becoming an employed physician for two or more years before becoming a full partner in a medical practice.

Currently, most physicians in training state they intend to become employed by a health system upon completion of their training, perhaps to bypass additional years of delay in full professional status in the setting of high levels of debt induced by the many years of medical education. What are the consequences for the physician and for society wrought by requiring such a prolonged period of training in order to achieve full professional status?

Among the most schooled professions, physicians achieve their full authority later in life than do all other professionals. This delay's impact on physicians personally and its impact on patients and the society they serve and by which they are supported needs to be carefully considered because much of the success or failure of healthcare delivery system transformation will require proficient physician leadership.

Physicians, who have delayed their full entry into adult professional roles longer than most of their contemporaries, have not necessarily been trained or selected adequately for leadership roles. Additionally, they have definite expectations about what this delay should ultimately bring to them, including high social status, adequate compensation, and meaningful work with appropriate autonomy in professional decision-making. When the implied social contract implicit in these expectations is not met, dysfunctional physician behavior may disrupt improvements in health system delivery.

The previously anticipated secure financial compensation at the end of their training is no longer certain for physicians who are experiencing declining reimbursements, loss of status, patients identifying alternative medications or non-traditional practitioners as equally qualified or valued, and consumerist pressures for improved access, results, and transparency. Physician-to-physician comparative data publicly accessible on the Internet adds competitive pressures that make compensation more dependent upon performance than on licensure in and of itself.

Despite its length, physician training does not include enough substantive attention to running a business, nor does it fully equip today's physicians for the evolution of healthcare that is occurring around them. Statistical process analysis, team-focused approaches to patient safety, and results-based, information-driven infrastructures upon which 21st-century healthcare systems will be based is not part of the skill set of the current physician workforce, nor is it part of the implicit bargain physicians thought they made with American society when they chose to spend their young adult years in the prolonged apprenticeship of medicine.

Cumulatively, these inherent challenges in the American medical education system, to some extent, stifle the opportunities for physicians to engage in leading the changes necessary for optimal patient care.

RIDING THE WAVES OF CHANGE

The medical community has faced a tremendous array of paradigm-shifting reforms leading up to our current position. The positive and negative transformative effects of alternative payment models, disruptive technology, and culture change have impacted the practice of medicine, its operating models, and its need for rapid adaption to ongoing innovation in the delivery system. Some of the forces of change impacting the medical profession include:

Emerging Technology — Artificial intelligence-generated point-of-care diagnostic tools, voice-recognition natural language processing, consumer-facing remote monitoring devices, 3D printing of human organs, blockchain-based solutions to the risk of security breaches, whole-genome sequencing life preventative health plans, and precision medicine-based oncology treatments are just a few of the emerging technologies that may vastly alter the traditional role clinicians play in the diagnostic and treatment of medical conditions in the next decade.

Some technologies that have been available for decades, such as telemedicine, rapidly accelerated during the pandemic, as regulatory barriers to remote access were removed for public safety reasons. The digital health revolution is poised to equalize the relationship between clinicians and patients and provide faster, more effective remedies for medical diseases. Nanotechnologies, robotics, augmented reality-assisted surgical procedures, and artificial intelligence algorithms are poised to redesign the entire healthcare experience.

Physicians may be more efficient as traditional workflows are automated, but the training needs of physicians may be vastly different from those currently supported by medical schools.

Integrated Behavioral Health Models — Behavioral health includes mental health and substance use disorders, life stressors and crises, stress-related physical symptoms, and health behaviors. In light of the prevalence of mental illnesses across all segments of the population and the interconnectedness with physical health, there is great interest in integrating mental health services with primary care services and especially with evolving efforts to expand the adoption of the patient-centered medical home model.[28]

In 2006, the IOM's Committee on Crossing the Quality Chasm identified four critical problems with the quality of mental/substance use (M/SU) care:

1. Failure to provide care consistent with existing scientific evidence;
2. Variations in care that occur when clear evidence on effective care is lacking;
3. Failure to provide any treatment for an M/SU illness or to address the risk factors associated with the development of these illnesses; and
4. Unsafe care.[29]

The fragmentation of behavioral health services results in the failure to provide an adequate safety net and infrastructure to treat M/SU issues experienced by certain patients has resulted in increased overall healthcare costs to payers, both private and governmental. For those seeking care for mental illness, limited access and insurance coverage for services, stigma, and discrimination are embedded in the overall infrastructure on a national level.[30]

Integrated behavioral health is part of a "whole-person" care model that is rapidly emerging as a principal component of high-quality care. Medical and behavioral health clinicians working together as a team to address a patient's health in a primary care setting has the advantage of better coordination and communication and improves access.[31]

Integrative Medicine — Integrative medicine (IM) may be considered complementary to or challenging of conventional medicine and can involve several types of treatments such as psycho-oncology, massage therapy, naturopathic medicine, acupuncture, Chinese herbal medicine, biofeedback, and nutraceuticals. Some of these approaches have been evaluated for their efficacy and safety, and providers who prescribe and utilize such interventions typically claim beneficial psychological and symptom improvement.[32]

Patients who experience adverse side effects that result from some conventional medical treatments, especially in the case of some cancer therapies and other chronic diseases, often turn to IM for alternative approaches to help lessen such side effects or in some cases to explore alternative interventions.

In 1998, the National Institute of Health (NIH) established the National Center for Complementary and Alternative Medicine (NCCAM).[33] This organization focuses on research on complementary and alternative medicine (CAM) to provide evidence as to the safety and efficacy of interventions that are adopted and used by practitioners, patients, and the general public for these types of treatments.

As the evidence base has grown, several academic medical centers[34] and hospital organizations have established centers and treatment services focused on IM and CAM, including Yale Integrative Medicine, Duke Integrative Medicine, Johns Hopkins Center for Complementary and Alternative Medicine, University of California San Francisco (UCSF) Osher Center for Integrative Medicine, and the Mayo Clinic.

Integrative medicine shifts the paradigm of traditional physician authority built upon 18th-century rationalism and 19th-century empiricism back to the alternative sources of authority built into the traditional shamanistic healer role. In Western cultural vernacular, alternative therapies emphasize the art rather than the science of medicine.

Patient-Centered Medical Homes — The patient-centered medical home (PCMH) is a model of care initially established in the field of pediatrics in the 1960s to provide care to children with complex illnesses. Initially conceived as an attempt at coordinating care for these children who often saw multiple and disconnected physicians, the American Academy of Pediatrics began advocating the concept of a medical home for all children, recognizing that fragmented care impacted all children.[35]

As accumulated research demonstrated that access to primary care improved outcomes and lowered costs, interest in the medical home model expanded to all patient populations. In 2007, the American College of Physicians, American Academy of Family Physicians, American Osteopathic Association, and the American Academy of Pediatrics adopted Joint Principles of the Patient-Centered Medical Home, recognizing that PCMHs should demonstrate processes and outcome performance in the following general areas:

1. **Personal physician:** Each patient has an ongoing relationship with a personal physician trained to provide first contact, continuous, and comprehensive care.
2. **Physician-directed team:** The personal physician leads a team of individuals at the practice level who collectively take responsibility for the ongoing care of patients.
3. **Whole-person orientation:** The personal physician is responsible for providing for all the patient's healthcare needs or taking responsibility for appropriately arranging care with other qualified professionals.
4. **Care coordination:** Care is coordinated and/or integrated across all elements of the complex healthcare system (e.g., subspecialty care, hospitals, home health agencies, nursing homes) and the patient's community (e.g., family, public, and private community-based services).
5. **Quality and safety:** These are hallmarks of the medical home.
6. **Enhanced access:** Access to care is available through systems such as open scheduling, expanded hours, and new options for communication between patients, their personal physician, and practice staff.
7. **Payment:** The payment structure appropriately recognizes the added value provided to patients who have a patient-centered medical home.[36]

The National Commission for Quality Assurance developed a PCMH recognition program in 2007 in which more than 95 organizations provide financial incentives, transformation support, care management, learning collaboratives, or maintenance of certification credit for participation in the accredited program.[37] Building on NCQA's earlier work, in 2015 Congress enacted the MACRA legislation, which explicitly linked recognized accredited patient-centered medical home programs with quality payments, including the NCQA's recognition program.

Patient Safety Movement — The 1999 release of the Institute of Medicine's *To Err is Human: Building a Safer Health System* was a bellwether moment, as it was the first time the impact and consequences of medical errors were quantified. The report acknowledged that more than 98,000 Americans were dying in hospitals from preventable causes.[38] The Office of Inspector General (OIG) indicated a decade later that the number of Medicare beneficiaries who had experienced an event in the hospital that contributed to their death had reached 180,000.[39]

Stakeholders from across the healthcare industry have collaborated in the research and development of safety policies, including the prioritization of non-technical skills such as teamwork, communication, and accountability and the development of various checklists and safety protocols from other industries, including crew resource management in aviation and process engineering.[40] Over the past 20 years, public policy and private efforts have included the Agency for Healthcare Research and Quality's (AHRQ) annual progress reports in monitoring patient safety improvement, the Joint Commission's addition of national patient safety goals to its credentialing process, the Institute for Healthcare Improvement's 100,000 lives campaign, the Associations of Academic Medical College's Integrating Quality Initiative, and the Affordable Care Act's Partnership for Patients. These are some of the ongoing efforts focused on eliminating medical harm from lapses in patient safety.

There has been progress, with the Department of Health and Human Services (DHHS) reporting that these initiatives had contributed to 125,000 fewer patients' deaths from hospital-acquired conditions between 2010 and 2015.[41] However, in the current COVID-19 pandemic, the catastrophic outcomes in long-term care settings and at the public health level experienced by the United States in comparison to other industrialized countries is the latest illustration of the complex nature of patient safety and the need to broaden our scope beyond the narrow focus of surgical operating rooms and intensive care units.

Payment Reform — The cost of healthcare services in America has grown exponentially over the past three decades, leading to legislative reform initiatives at both federal and state levels as consumers, employers, and the government attempt to exert control over the escalating cost of care. While cost increases are partially fueled by advancements in medical technologies, pharmacotherapy, and research, they are partially a result of waste, fraud, and misuse of medical therapies incentivized by the volume-based fee-for-service systems.

At the federal level, the DHHS, OIG, Centers for Medicare and Medicaid Services (CMS), and the Department of Justice are escalating enforcement of fraud and abuse [42] and anti-trust laws, employing new methods such as the CMS Recovery Audit Contractor program, adopting the Correct Coding Initiative in CMS programs, and intensifying the bundling of codes for previously separately reimbursed services.

Despite these ongoing regulatory approaches to cost control, healthcare costs have continued to rise, prompting recognition of the need to reform fee-for-service payment models across the political spectrum. Embedded in the 2010 Patient Protection and Affordable Care Act was the establishment of the Center for Medicare and Medicaid Innovation (CMMI) to "test innovative payment and delivery system models that show important promise for maintaining or improving the quality of care in Medicare, Medicaid, and the Children's Health Insurance Program (CHIP) while slowing the rate of growth in program costs."[43]

The 2015 Medicare Access and CHIP Reauthorization Act (MACRA) augmented these federal efforts with language to establish the Physician-Focused Payment Model Technical Advisory Committee to review and assess physician-focused payment models (PFPMs) based on stakeholder proposals submitted to the committee with criteria based on improving care or reducing costs.[44]

Quality Improvement — The roots of the clinical quality improvement movement go back as far as Ignaz Semmelweis's 19th-century efforts to promote handwashing in medical care. His recognition that quality could be improved by measurement still holds true and remains the crucial strategy for successful process improvement.

Physician leadership is recognized as an essential element in successful healthcare quality improvement efforts, along with infrastructural support and prioritization of healthcare quality within the culture of the organization. Increasingly, reimbursement rates for physician services are tied to the demonstration of clinical quality through pay-for-performance programs with commercial payers and governmental payers.

Key provisions focused on quality in the Patient Protection and Affordable Care Act include the establishment of the Patient-Centered Outcomes Research Institute (PCORI) to accelerate comparative effectiveness efforts and the implementation of Accountable Care Organizations (ACOs) intended to guide the healthcare industry towards payment models that incentivize high quality and coordination of care.[45] The near-unanimous congressional passage of the MACRA legislation in 2015 established the requirement of quality of care reporting for physician payments across the board.

In 2001, the IOM's call in *Crossing the Quality Chasm* to develop a 21st-century healthcare system asserted that a new system could improve, not just alter, healthcare by refocusing on the patient. The IOM declared that our healthcare system should aim to be safe, timely, efficient, effective, equitable, and patient-centered. [46] These six aims have served as the underpinning foundation for many care delivery reform initiatives, research programs, and other transformational initiatives that are underway or have occurred across the country over the past decade.

Sadly, the majority of physicians in American have not read *Crossing the Quality Chasm* or the IOM's 1999 report *To Err Is Human* that focused on improving patient safety. The 2011 IOM report calling for leadership in nursing in the new health system ironically challenges physicians to intensify their leadership role in order to appropriately remain relevant in the national agenda.[47]

The proposed agenda from the IOM Committee on Quality of Healthcare in America calls on healthcare leaders to:

- Design and implement more effective organizational support processes.
- Create a national environment that fosters and rewards improvement.
- Commit to a national statement of purpose and the six aims for improvement.
- Adopt principles to guide the design of care processes.
- Identify priority conditions to provide resources to stimulate innovation.
- The key tenets of this agenda have influenced many of the policy decisions of private and governmental payers over the past decade and are radically changing the culture of American medicine.[48]

As it was proposed two decades ago, this agenda led to the commitment to a national statement of purpose that is apparent through the multi-year effort that brought about the Affordable Care Act in 2010 and MACRA in 2015 that prioritized focusing the agenda on national healthcare redesign. The IOM's generation of a national dialogue endorsing an environment that rewards improvement has catalyzed the move away from a volume-driven reimbursement system to one that is driven by and pays for performance and delivery of value-added services.

Twenty-two years after the IOM publication, the healthcare community is still working to implement initiatives to meet the IOM's goals. What will it take for physician leaders to achieve these objectives fully in the 21st century?

In 2012, the Oliver Wyman Healthcare Innovation Center released a series of white papers describing the three waves of transformation about to engulf the healthcare industry between 2010 and 2025.[49] Wave 1 would focus on patient-centered care and population health management. Wave 2 would focus more on consumer engagement and the quantified self. Wave 3 would bring forth the science of prevention built upon affordable genomic data and mobile apps navigating a person's health profile.

The innovation center posited Wave 1 as occurring between 2010 and 2016, when healthcare moved from a physician-centered to a patient-focused model, with transactional, fragmented care replaced by care team management, convenient 24/7 access, and evidence-based standards extinguishing unexplained variations in quality.

Wave 2, which presumably crested 2014 to 2020, informed shared decision-making with highly engaged, empowered consumers who are socially connected with virtual mobile, anytime access to care would become normative. Wave 3, 2018 to 2025, described the science of prevention, where monitoring and prevention, a genome-linked life plan, and personalized therapies, 100% accurate diagnoses, and life, social, and ethics competencies were integrated with medical competencies.

Looking back, some of this vision was accurate. PCMHs, ACOs, telemedicine, smart-phone health apps, evidence-based medicine, shared medical decision-making, and $100 genomes have been established. The Moderna COVID-19 vaccine, built upon the new CRISPR-based genomic technologies, was fully developed by January 2020 and deployed worldwide within a year.

Yet, the healthcare delivery system of 2021 is anything but perfect. Waves 4, 5, and 6 of transformation are already underway, while the first three waves of change have yet to mature.

The task for physicians is to learn how to lead as these waves keep crashing. Many people believe the nation's physicians are ill-equipped to manage the tsunami of change engulfing the healthcare system. Physicians must be prepared to collaboratively lead in an environment that is changing faster than any we have ever had to lead in before. Physicians face challenges that range from burnout to pandemic fatigue, poorly designed electronic health records, reduction in power and clinical autonomy, unfunded regulatory requirements, payment models in transition, institutional racism, gender bias, outmoded training, and six-figure student loan debt. These challenges, by their very nature, cannot be adequately addressed within the context of the traditional authoritarian, paternalistic physician role.

Twenty-first-century healthcare can be physician-led and patient-centered. It can be team-based, collaborative, technically advanced, and relevant in complex adaptive systems. But physicians will need a new toolset that engenders resilience and inculcates proactive change management behaviors. Keep reading.

REFERENCES

1. Lincoln A. Annual Message to Congress. Concluding Remarks. Accessed online at http://www.abrahamlincolnonline.org/lincoln/speeches/congress.htm.

2. Specter M. How Anthony Fauci Became America's Doctor. *The New Yorker. April 20, 2020.* https://web.archive.org/web/20200413235133/https://www.newyorker.com/magazine/2020/04/20/how-anthony-fauci-became-americas-doctor.

3. Cox CE. From Heroes to Humans: How Doctors Found Their Voices in 2020. tctMD December 21, 2020. www.tctmd.com/news/heroes-humans-how-doctors-found-their-voices-2020.

4. Murphy B. New AMA President: As Physician-Heroes We Will Confront Challenges. AMA. June 7, 2020. www.ama-assn.org/house-delegates/special-meeting/new-ama-president-physician-heroes-we-will-confront-challenges.

5. Noack R, Mellen R. Around the World, Health Officials Face Death Threats Amid Pandemic. *The Washington Post. September 14, 2020.* www.washingtonpost.com/world/2020/09/14/coronavirus-death-threats-global-health-officials.

6. Drummond D. Stop Calling Doctors Heroes and Saints: The Case Against Altruism. Medscape. November 24, 2020. www.medscape.com/viewarticle/941446.

7. Drummond D. Physician Burnout: Its Origin, Symptoms, and Five Main Causes. *Fam Pract Manag. 2015 Sep-Oct (5)42-47.* https://www.aafp.org/fpm/2015/0900/p42.html.

8. New Health Guide. Highest Suicide Rate by Profession. New Health Guide. 2021. www.newhealthguide.org/Highest-Suicide-Rate-By-Profession.html.

9. Hartzband P, Groopman J. Physician Burnout, Interrupted. *NEJM. 2020; 382:2485–2487.* www.nejm.org/doi/full/10.1056/NEJMp2003149?query=RP#.XqxYUMVNeNE.twitter.

10. Kamal R, McDermott D, Ramirez G, Cox C. How Has U.S. Spending on Healthcare Changed Over Time? Peterson-KFF Health System Tracker. December 2020. www.healthsystemtracker.org/chart-collection/u-s-spending-healthcare-changed-time/#item-usspendingovertime_10.

11. Committee for a Responsible Federal Budget. American Health Care: Health Spending and the Federal Budget. Committee for a Responsible Federal Budget. May 16, 2018. www.crfb.org/papers/american-health-care-health-spending-and-federal-budget

12. Statista. U.S. National Health Expenditure as Percent of GDPA from 1960 to 2020. Statista.com. September 8, 2021. www.statista.com/statistics/184968/us-health-expenditure-as-percent-of-gdp-since-1960.

13. Silko AM, Truffer CJ, Keehan SP, Poisal JA, Clemens MK, Madison AJ. National Health Spending Projections: The Estimated Impact of Reform Through 2019. *Health Aff (Millwood).* 2010;29(10):1933-1941.

14. Tolbert J, Orgera K, Damico A. Key Facts About the Uninsured Population. Kaiser Family Foundation Issue Brief. November 6, 2020. www.kff.org/uninsured/issue-brief/key-facts-about-the-uninsured-population.

15. McDermott D, Cox C, Rudowitz R, Garfield R. How Has the Pandemic Affected Health Coverage in the U.S.? Kaiser Family Foundation. December 9, 2020. www.kff.org/policy-watch/how-has-the-pandemic-affected-health-coverage-in-the-u-s.

16. Institute of Medicine, Committee on Quality of Healthcare in America. *To Err Is Human.* Washington, DC: National Academies Press; 2000.

17. Rodziewicz TL, Houseman B, Hipskind JE. Medical Errof Reduction and Prevention. StatsPearls [Internet]. August 6, 2021. www.ncbi.nlm.nih.gov/books/NBK499956/#:~:text=Medical%20errors%20cost%20approximately%20%2420,%2C%20falls%2C%20and%20healthcare%20technology.

18. Johns Hopkins Medicine. Study Suggests Medical Errors Now Third Leading Cause of Death in the U.s. News Release. May 3, 2016. www.hopkinsmedicine.org/news/media/releases/study_suggests_medical_errors_now_third_leading_cause_of_death_in_the_us

19. The Physicians Foundation. 2018 Survey of America's Physicians: Practice Patterns and Perspectives. The Physicians Foundation. 2018. https://physiciansfoundation.org/wp-content/uploads/2018/09/physicians-survey-results-final-2018.pdf.

20. Magner L. *A History of Medicine*. New York: Marcel Dekker, Inc.;1992, pp. 1-15.

21. Starr P. *The Social Transformation of American Medicine*. New York, NY: Harper Collins;1982, p. 3.

22. Starr, p. 4.

23. Starr, p. 27.

24. Institute of Medicine, Board on Health Sciences Policy, Committee of Understanding and Eliminating Racial and Ethnic Disparities in Healthcare, *Unequal Treatment: Confronting Racial and Ethnic Disparities in Healthcare. Washington, DC: National Academies Press; 2009.*

25. Klass P. *A Good Time to Be Born: How Science and Public Health Gave Children a Future. New York, NY: W.W. Norton and Company; 2020, p. 127.*

26. Starr, p. 4.

27. Starr, p. 446.

28. Hogan MF, Sederer LI, Smith TE, Nossel IR. Making Room for Mental Health in the Medical Home. *Prev Chronic Dis* 2010;7(6).

29. Institute of Medicine, Committee on Quality of Health Care in America. *Crossing the Quality Chasm: Adaptation to Mental Health and Addictive Disorders. Improving the Quality of Healthcare for Mental and Substance-Use Conditions: Quality Chasm Series.* Washington, DC: National Academies Press; 2006, p. 141.

30. Institute of Medicine, *Improving the Quality of Healthcare for Mental and Substance-Use Conditions: Quality Chasm Series,* pp. xi-xii.

31. Agency for Healthcare Research and Quality. What Is Integrated Behavioral Health? https://integrationacademy.ahrq.gov/about/integrated-behavioral-health.

32. Diehl V. The Bridge Between Patient and Doctor: The Shift from CAM to Integrative Medicine. *Hematology Am Soc Hematol Educ Program.* 2009;320-5.

33. National Center for Complementary and Alternative Medicine (NCCAM). Strategic Plans and Reports. http://nccam.nih.gov/about/plans/2011.

34. Millet J. Progress in Complementary and Alternative Medicine Research. *Yale J Biol Med.* 2010; 83(3):127-9.

35. O'Dell ML. What Is a Patient-Centered Medical Home? *Mo Med. 2016; 113(4):301-4.* www.ncbi.nlm.nih.gov/pmc/articles/PMC6139911.

36. Patient-Centered Primary Care Collaborative. Defining the Medical Home. www.pcpcc.org/about/medical-home.

37. NCQA. Patient-Centered Medical Home. NCQA. www.ncqa.org/programs/health-care-providers-practices/patient-centered-medical-home-pcmh.

38. Institute of Medicine. *To Err Is Human: Building a Safer Health System.* Washington, DC: Institute of Medicine; 1999.

39. Patient Safety Movement. Vision: Achieve ZERO Preventable Patient Harm and Death Across the Globe by 2030. https://patientsafetymovement.org/about.

40. Lark ME, Kirkpatrick K, Chung CK. Patient Safety Movement: History and Future Directions. *J Hand Surg Am. 2018;43(2):174-8.* www.ncbi.nlm.nih.gov/pmc/articles/PMC5808589.

41. Agency for Healthcare Research and Quality. National Scorecard on Rates of Hospital-Acquired Conditions 2010 to 2015: Interim Data from National Efforts to Make Healthcare Safer. www.ahrq.gov/hai/pfp/2015-interim.html.

42. U.S. Department of Health and Human Services Office of the Inspector General. *A Roadmap for New Physicians. Avoiding Medicare and Medicaid Fraud and Abuse.* pp. 2-8. Washington, DC: U.S. Department of Health and Human Services Office of the Inspector General. http://oig.hhs.gov/compliance/physician-education/roadmap_web_version.pdf.

43. Centers for Medicare & Medicaid Services. Where Innovation Is Happening. cms.org. www.innovation.cms.gov.

44. Centers for Medicare & Medicaid Services. Innovation Models. cms.org. https://innovation.cms.gov/innovation-models/pfpms.

45. Marjoua Y, Bozic K. Brief History of Quality Movement in US Healthcare. *Curr Rev Musculoskeletal Med. 2012 Dec; 5(4):265-73.* www.ncbi.nlm.nih.gov/pmc/articles/PMC3702754.

46. Institute of Medicine, Committee on Quality of Healthcare in America. Building Organizational Support for Change. In *Crossing the Quality Chasm: A New Health System for the 21st Century.* Washington, DC: National Academies Press; 2001, pp. 5-6.

47. Institute of Medicine. Committee on the Robert Wood Johnson Foundation Initiative on the Future of Nursing, at the Institute of Medicine. Summary. In *The Future of Nursing: Leading Change, Advancing Health.* Washington, DC: National Academies Press; 2011, p. 8.

48. Institute of Medicine, *Crossing the Quality Chasm: A New Health System for the 21st Century.* Washington, DC: National Academies Press; 2001, p. 34.

49. OliverWyman. The Volume-to-Value Revolution. https://www.oliverwyman.com/our-expertise/insights/2012/nov/the-volume-to-value-revolution.html.

CHAPTER 1: WHERE WE STAND
Leadership Implications and Health Policy Considerations

Leadership Implications:

1. Recognize the extraordinary impact the global pandemic has had on the physician workforce, with the traditional heroic stereotype engendering burnout and the underinvestment in public health indicting the traditional assumptions of the healthcare delivery system by failing to contain the pandemic.
2. Evaluate how impending demographic and technology changes will challenge contemporary medical professionalism.

Health Policy Considerations:

1. When developing workable national healthcare policies, determine the relevance of historical and contemporary medical professional culture to the waves of technical and social change impacting healthcare delivery.
2. Juxtapose emerging technology innovations, demographic trends, and social change to model clinical care models efficient and effective enough to improve patient access and outcomes in the next two decades.

CHAPTER 2

Powershift and Teambuilding

When opportunities in a profession change, so does the profession.[1]

Paul Starr

Traditionally, physicians have been honored with high status and respect. Death and disease are a universal part of human experience; those whose role it is to relieve suffering are valued highly in all cultures. As the 18th-century scientific revolution advanced the tools of care with medical breakthroughs that relieved physical suffering, the role of the healer focused less on the relief of spiritual suffering. The 19th and 20th centuries saw surgeries performed with anesthesia, a rapid deceleration in death associated with childbirth, and infectious diseases combatted with antibiotics. As the professionals who controlled the means to new treatments and interventions, physicians assumed a prestigious social status that was typically accompanied by a great level of wealth.

However, by the last quarter of the 20th century, the continuously shifting healthcare ecosystem impacted physicians' social status, authority, and prestige. Powershifts have included broader income disparities between physicians performing procedures focused on diagnosis and management; loss of professional independence necessitated by being part of integrated health delivery systems to have access to technology and teams; increased regulatory burden; and high business transaction costs caused by payers using managed care techniques to control costs.

Futurist Alvin Toffler understood power to be based on three components: knowledge, wealth, and force. He posited that knowledge is the most potent form of power in our society because we live in a knowledge-based civilization.[2] Within Toffler's framework, the rise of professional physician power is the result of control of medical knowledge, and the shifts in power result from changes in the span of control of medical knowledge.

One driver of this shift has been the acceleration of information technology in expanding access to medical knowledge and in the exponential growth of medical knowledge itself. Technological innovations have re-balanced asymmetries of information access between physicians and patients along the continuums of care.

To operate with maximum efficiency, the highly complex healthcare delivery system requires integrated knowledge management in a patient-centric context. With this technology-induced change comes a transformation in the culture and a necessarily fresh approach to relationships with peers and teams, new collaborative problem solving, shared leadership, and shared decision-making. This cultural transformation is a shift in power traditionally held by physicians in their professional role from one focused on authority and autonomy to one focused on leadership and collaboration.

Four forces affecting the locus of control in the healthcare delivery system will continue to transform the medical profession.

First, the physician-patient relationship will continue to undergo significant changes. In 1982, Paul Starr identified three claims to be met for the "*legitimation of professional authority*":

1. Knowledge and competence are validated by peers.
2. The validated knowledge and competence rest on a rational and scientific basis; and
3. The professional's judgment and advice are structured around relevant values.[3]

The exponential expansion and availability of information brought about through the Internet permit patients' direct access to medical information while also expanding evidence-based medicine with clinical decision support. As patients and physicians interact in an information-rich world, the peer-validated knowledge and competence of professional authority are challenged by the open, consumerist culture of the web.

Second, physicians' social and structural authority with peers and clinician team members has been impacted by electronic health records and other health information technology solutions. The balance of power and responsibilities in the care delivery process has shifted. One example is the rise of pharmacists' provision of comprehensive medication management. Integration of pharmacist-led medication management has improved patient care through medication reconciliation, comprehensive medication reviews, medication adherence promotion, and chronic disease management.[4]

Similarly, population health management analytic technology permits non-physician healthcare professionals to identify cohorts of patients in a population with specific medical conditions or risk factors and address them in ways not dependent on traditional clinic interactions. These examples illustrate how a team approach to chronic management is facilitated by the multi-user access of the electronic health record.

Third, the authority and autonomy of physicians in their clinical role does not necessarily translate to similar authority in the healthcare organization in which they work, as the industry continues its transition away from a cottage industry culture to one built upon corporate governance and infrastructure. The governance of corporations depends on boards of directors and professional managers. The shift in power created by the corporatization of medicine reinforces the need for business acumen and education in management if physicians are to have a seat in the executive suite and boardroom.

Fourth, healthcare industry economic trends over the past half-century directly contribute to physicians' loss of traditional autonomy. These trends include changes to the principal-agent relationship, reduction in monopolistic power, and changes in the healthcare labor market. The principal agent relationship occurs when one person is allowed to make decisions on behalf of another person.

Historically, the physician-patient relationship had principal agent components, with physicians making decisions on behalf of their patients, sometimes with little input from the patients themselves. Over the past few decades, legal constructs such as living wills, designated healthcare power of attorney, and informed consent have replaced "doctor knows best" power constructs.

Shared decision-making equalizes the power relationship even more. As other medical professionals expand the scope of their licenses, diagnostic, management, and treatment capabilities are shared with other healthcare professionals. The ongoing expansion of the medical and surgical specialties and the expansion of the healthcare labor market to include new professionals such as advance practice providers, clinical pharmacists, physical therapists, respiratory therapists, clinical psychologists, licensed clinical social workers, and clinical nurse managers differentiate the healthcare labor force into a highly skilled market with far greater scope and scale.

In light of the complexity of the U.S. healthcare system and changing global economic landscape over the past quarter-century, these trends have contributed to shifts in the physician's authority and control over healthcare services. While health reform initiatives are developed and approved for application at federal and state levels, the implementation of new policy occurs at the micro-level in regional integrated delivery systems, multispecialty groups, physician hospital organizations, and clinically integrated networks.

Consumer-facing models of care enabled by technology, retail clinics, social networking, asynchronous information exchange via patient portals, remote monitoring, and smartphone apps disrupt established healthcare delivery models upon which physician power was historically based.

A great deal of status anxiety among physicians is driven by the impact of these four forces on professional power, so continuation of physician leadership within the evolving industry requires physicians to take on new roles and skills that transcend traditional authority and are consilient with the new needs of patients as empowered and informed consumers.

FORCE ONE: THE NEW PHYSICIAN-PATIENT RELATIONSHIP

Consumer sovereignty is affected by the advantage physicians have in the asymmetries of information and medical knowledge with patients. Internet access has altered but not eliminated this asymmetry. Patients still rely on their physicians to diagnose and recommend treatments based on their clinical experience, which inculcates an intrinsic compact in the relationship. This compact is based on the patient's trust in professional judgment and ethical behavior.

In 2002, studies in six countries on four continents revealed that the citizens of all countries viewed the patient-physician relationship as second in importance to family relationships. The patient-physician relationship scored higher than spiritual, financial, and co-worker relationships. While the relationship has always been highly valued, it is certainly not static. In all countries studied, the relationship was rapidly evolving. Authoritarian, paternalistic relationships in which "doctor says" and "patient does " are increasingly in the minority. They have been replaced by collaborative partnerships with 50/50 decision-making and advisor relationships in which the physician serves as a resource and guide, but patients take responsibility for decisions on their own healthcare.[5]

Since the 1990s, the healthcare and medically related information available to the general public via web-based technology has grown exponentially, bringing about a shift in the balance of information accessible to consumers. Increased transparency of cost and quality information on physician and hospital services is resulting in a stronger base of patient knowledge. Early consumer-directed tools such as Vitals (www. vitals.com) and Health

Grades (www.healthgrades.com), and the Department of Health and Human Services Hospital Compare website (https://www.cms.gov/Medicare/Quality-Initiatives-Patient-Assessment-Instruments/HospitalQualityInits/HospitalCompare) emerged in the first decade of the 21st century and have been joined by thousands more.

The rise of social media platforms has created communities focused on various health and medical concerns, with information exchange of varying quality and not always based on sound medical science. Understanding the difference between patients and consumers is important. As Jeff Margolis explains, "People use the terms patient and consumer interchangeably, but they are not the same. Patients receive care, and consumers make choices. Engaged patients adhere to or comply with a treatment regimen given to them by healthcare professionals, while engaged consumers are accountable for their overall health status and the costs of achieving that health status."[6] Patient portals, personal health records, mobile-centric health apps, and wearable devices are some of the emerging technologies that are accelerating the transformation of passive patients into engaged consumers.

One of the most significant changes to emerge in the past two decades in the physician-patient relationship has been increased shared decision-making. The Institute of Medicine's objective for patient-centered care cannot be achieved without a shift in asymmetries of information. Godolphin notes that there are several strategies for physicians to engage and barriers to overcome in shared decision-making situations with patients:

- Understanding the patient's preferences, values, beliefs, and expectations.
- Establishing partnership approaches/philosophies to relationships with patients that position themselves as a mentor and advisor when needed in the patient's clinical decision-making process.
- Helping patients develop and recognize choices in meeting their medical care needs. (While the gap in information asymmetries has closed, the physician's clinical training and experience will always hold value beyond what the lay members of society can absorb.)
- Planning to devote more time to shared decision-making processes with patients.
- Recognizing and respecting the patient's decisions.[7]

For the physician leader, this shift in power in the relationship with patients has organizational and managerial implications. Following practice guidelines or meeting requirements for administering services at hospitals may require certain physician behaviors and communications to adhere to established risk management, quality, or safety policies. Integrating shared decision-making into practice policies will be a cultural shift for every organization.

FORCE TWO: HEALTH INFORMATION TECHNOLOGY

The perpetual influx of innovative technologies into the healthcare delivery process simultaneously offers ongoing medical advances and personal challenges for practicing physicians. Surgical robotics, precision pharmacology, genomics and proteomics, diagnostic nanotechnologies, artificial intelligence, and advanced analytics will continue to deliver new capabilities and power to the physician community while simultaneously challenging the capacity of physicians to adapt to the ever-increasing complexity of their practice environment. In 1982, Starr noted that technology increased physician power:

> . . . the most influential explanation for the structure of American medicine gives primary emphasis to scientific and technological change and specifically attributes the rise of medical authority to the improved therapeutic competence of physicians.[8]

In years after Starr's analysis, not only have the advancements made through technological change enabled many of the industry's breakthroughs and life-saving accomplishments, but they also challenged physicians' professional control. Robotic surgery changed the capital requirements of hospitals, decreased recovery time for patients, and required new technical skills for surgeons. Likewise, population management strategies dependent on "Big Data" information technology in the community setting altered medical practice's historical facility-based episodic business model.

Just as patients have gained access to better information to improve their own decision-making, so too have the tools improved for physicians to support clinical diagnosis recommendations and orders for better-quality medical care. Using the best knowledge to identify what to do and how to make it part of routine practice may appear obvious. Still, studies indicate it takes up to 15 years for medical knowledge to become incorporated into routine medical practice.

Unexplained variation in clinical practice is prevalent throughout clinical settings to the extent that the integration of content and context is seldom ideal. Evidence-based medicine provides the practicing physician a bridge between science and bedside application that can serve as a pathway to transition practice guidelines to a more precision-based and scientifically rigorous methodology.

Unintended Adverse Consequences with Computerized Physician Order Entry Implementation
A study of five community and academic hospitals with significant computerized physician order entry systems implemented. Data collection occurred between August 2004 and April 2005 with extensive analysis by the research team that ensued in the following years. In the study, the team identified nine unintended adverse consequences:

1. More/new work for clinicians
2. Workflow issues
3. Never-ending system demands
4. Paper persistence
5. Changes in communication patterns and practices
6. Emotions
7. New kinds of errors
8. Changes in power structure
9. Overdependence on technology

Figure 1.

The use of evidence-based medicine should ensure that patient care adheres to clinical best practices and improves the health of communities. However, with evidence-based medicine and evidence-based management come perceived threats to autonomy and control in clinical decision-making, difficulty accessing the evidence base, and difficulty differentiating useful and accurate evidence from that which is inaccurate or inapplicable. Integrating evidence-based medicine practices into clinical guidelines requires physicians who can draw upon the evidence to improve the quality of care being delivered.[9]

The introduction of new technology within the clinical work environment always alters processes and has unintended consequences. A classic example of unintentional consequences is the 2006 study by Campbell, Sittig, Ash, and colleagues identifying a set of nine unintended adverse consequences that result from the introduction of computerized physician order entry systems. The authors note an unintended power structure shift from physicians to others based on their loss of control over information.[10]

A deeper understanding of the technologies' role in healthcare power shifts is the interactive sociotechnical analysis (ISTA) introduced by Harrison and Koppel in 2007.[11] Computerized provider order entry and other health information technology systems all involve transforming the clinical workflow processes within organizations as they are implemented. Throughout the process of design, test, implementation, and eventual future-state use of a new application, clinician, ancillary, and administrative team members are engaged with physicians to ensure that benefits are realized from the new tools to meet goals for improving outcomes, cost, quality, and safety of patient care.

Harrison and Koppel indicate that, throughout this process, relationships and communication are impacted by the dynamics involved with changes in workflow and the new systems. New triggers, alerts, and in some cases, workarounds[12] can emerge that inadvertently result in shifts of roles and actions that can impact quality and safety in patient care operations. Harrison's and Koppel's ISTA model can be applied to manage resources needed to accommodate new workflows, approvals, communication patterns, and roles of various professionals in the healthcare system.

The shift in control of information brought on by health information technology improvements has led to an increase in leadership roles held by nurses and other non-physicians in the care delivery process and administration of healthcare organizations. Nurses make up the largest segment of the healthcare workforce. As their responsibilities have grown to accommodate the needs of delivering patient-centered care, academic initiatives are focused on strengthening the education level of the national nursing workforce. As a result, a growing number of nursing leaders are working in partnership with physicians to redesign the healthcare delivery system and processes.[13] Several factors are driving this change:

- The social architecture and fabric of healthcare organizations have changed. Nurses are increasingly being called upon to shape health policy, implement new systems, and serve as change agents throughout the healthcare ecosystem.

- Health information technology tools have increased the need for shared responsibilities in managing health information at the patient and population levels.

- The patient population continues to increase through demographic and socioeconomic changes that will drive the need for additional collaborative clinical leadership in managing care delivery programs and organizations.[14]

Team-based care is inevitable and crucial for improving patient outcomes as technology continues to accelerate changes in the healthcare delivery system. Team-based healthcare includes collaboration among team members and the patient and family, shared goals across healthcare settings, and coordinated, high-quality, patient-centered care.[15] However, who and how leadership and authority are distributed in healthcare teams remain controversial. The American Medical Association supports legislation that maintains the authority of physicians in patient care and advocates for physician-led team models,[16] but with the worldwide shortages of primary care physicians, non-physician healthcare professionals are taking an increasing role in leading teams in order to maintain access to primary care across the world.

Artificial intelligence-driven algorithms may supersede the seven years of medical training traditionally required to train a primary care physician and permit the design of high-functioning healthcare teams built upon non-physician professionals with a different skill set and training from that provided by medical personnel schools. Regardless of authority structure, team-based care requires shared accountability for patient care and timely information that is shared comprehensively among the team members. [17] Improvements in health information technology can optimize team-based care.

FORCE THREE: FROM COTTAGE INDUSTRY TO CORPORATE MEDICINE

Even into the last decades of the 20th century, most physicians operated in a cottage industry environment built on small, physician-owned independent practices operated independently but collaboratively with one another as voluntary members of community hospital medical staff. Alternative practice models, such as physicians employed by hospitals or independent group practices (such as Kaiser Permanente), gradually became more dominant. The benefits of the integrated practice models include access to more predictable, standardized compensation and benefits, access to better technology, and more favorable reimbursement from payers based on the ability of larger medical groups to negotiate rates with payers.

By 2018, about 31.4% of physicians identified as independent practice owners. The Physicians Foundation and Merritt Hawkins survey in 2018 indicated that the hospital employment model now dominates the industry, with younger physicians preferring employment to independent practice ownership.[18] As an economic necessity, the era of smaller independent physician practices is coming to a close. As the Physicians Foundation Merritt Hawkins survey indicates:

> "These data suggest that the independent practice model is under pressure in a healthcare system increasingly dominated by large, integrated organizations, whether hospital systems, large medical groups, corporations or insurance companies. . . . All of these entities typically implement the employed physician model to achieve the standardized physician compensation formulas, electronic health records, quality measures and treatment guidelines necessary in an era of global, quality-based payments and population health management."[19]

The COVID-19 pandemic has put added pressure on independent medical practices that are highly dependent on the steady flow of fee-for-service revenue, which dropped abruptly at the onset of the pandemic.[20] Employment by a corporate entity may offer physicians more stable compensation, improved benefits, and relative safety navigating the challenges of a rapidly evolving industry.

Some of the new insurance-owned practices, such as United Health Care's OptumCare Medical Group, have expanded substantially during the pandemic, with large independent medical groups such as Caramount Medical Group in New York and Oregon Medical Group joining the more than 35,000 other providers that now make Optum the largest medical practice in the country.

With this industry transition to corporate structures, the importance of having physicians operating in the governance and leadership of the new healthcare corporate institutions has become a priority. Many hospital-owned medical practices and payer-owned medical practices have minimal experience with physician leadership in the C-suite or board room. In academic medicine, however, the traditional positions of power continue to be held by physicians. The physician's knowledge, skills, and ethical responsibilities have emerged as essential to the spectrum of other organizational types operating in the healthcare ecosystem. Companies ranging from biotechnology start-ups to managed-care organizations and government agencies are calling upon physicians to take leadership to create sustainable healthcare institutions.

FORCE FOUR: HEALTHCARE MACROECONOMICS

The pandemic has worsened the looming insolvency of the Medicare Trust Fund. The Congressional Budget Office projects that in the wake of the coronavirus pandemic, the Medicare Hospital Insurance Trust Fund, which pays for hospital, nursing facility, home health, and hospice services provided under traditional Medicare and Medicare Advantage plans, will become insolvent in 2024, two years sooner than predicted.[21]

Given these projections, it is noteworthy that MedPAC's top reason for the growth in healthcare spending over the past four decades is advances in technology. In that dynamic, the physician's role as an autonomous decision-maker for the utilization of such technologies will continue to be challenged. The exorbitantly high increase in costs will continue to push a regulatory response and a reform agenda such as value-based purchasing, bundled payment systems, across-the-board cuts in fees, and alternative payment models. Thus, physician leadership must understand the impact that economic trends will have upon the profession from a comprehensive standpoint.

Changes to the principal-agent relationship. Agency theory formulates the concept of the principal (patient) and agent (physician) relationship that should be the foundation of patient-centered decisions and programs. The economics of health insurance benefits structure and intrinsic perverse financial incentives present across the spectrum of fee-for-service, capitation, and pay-for-performance reimbursement models, translate into *moral hazard* that impacts the physician-patient relationship directly.[22] The inherent moral hazard of *supplier-induced demand*[23] has given rise to the importance of pay-for-performance reimbursement systems and other value-based purchasing programs.

Shared decision-making may mitigate the risks of supplier-induced demand, but it will not control the moral hazard of overutilization by insured patients without some market-dependent cost-shifting to patients from third-party payers, or provider-based global payment systems such as ACOs in which providers take on the risk of overutilization and underutilization.

Reduction in monopolistic power. The monopolistic power once held by physicians has been eliminated by their need for access to capital to provide technology-based care and the lack of ability of independent physicians to take on substantial business risk. As the holders of capital and risk, respectively, large health systems and insurance companies operate in an environment of scrutiny by the Department of Justice and the Federal Trade Commission, which monitor the pro-competitive and anti-competitive effects of mergers and acquisitions of physicians' practices.

Additionally, increased consumer awareness of the quality and cost of services provided by physicians has developed over the past 20 years as a result of online access to data, consumer-rating websites, and regulatory transparency efforts. Combined, these issues have resulted in a decrease in the monopolistic power once held by the physician profession. Insured patients understand that they have more choices and, therefore, can work in partnership with physicians to make better economic decisions about the management of their care. The changes coming through federal and state health reforms will affect the competitive landscape for medical services throughout every region of the country.

Changes in labor market for physicians and nurses. In the late 1990s, enrollments for certain physician specialties in medical schools started to decline. General surgery, general internal medicine, and family practice have seen dramatic declines. The increase in both status and life-long income for procedure-based specialists over generalists, along with the high cost of financing a medical education, created a precipitous drop-off in the primary care workforce. Simultaneously there are significant shortages forecasted to occur nationally in the nursing workforce.[24]

In light of this projection, in 2009, the American Recovery and Reinvestment Act (ARRA) identified a number of programs to increase educational funding to support the growth of both junior and advanced nursing degrees.[25] These workforce trends have caused changes in strategy for how best to deliver optimal patient care services throughout regions of the country where the workforce shortages have had the most dramatic impacts.

From the perspective of physician leaders, the shifts in power and autonomy in both clinical decision-making and administrative matters have been impacted more from the standpoint of necessity brought on by changes in the labor force than by any other phenomena.

HEALTHCARE IS NOW A TEAM SPORT

Optimal team-based healthcare is associated with improvement in patient outcomes and physician well-being. A healthcare team is a group of individuals who work together interdependently and coordinate their actions to prevent or treat disease and promote health. Team-based models of care endeavor to meet patient needs and preferences with active patient engagement, and encourage all healthcare professionals to function to the full extent of their education, certification, and experience.

Multidisciplinary team-based care is associated with better performance on healthcare quality measures and is cost-effective. Teamwork can prevent adverse patient outcomes and is thus an important part of patient safety efforts. Preliminary studies of clinician burnout indicate that high-performing teams can reduce clinician burnout.

As innovations in delivery models and reimbursement models emerge, the healthcare industry will experience further shifts in the social power structures, levels of autonomy, and control that affect the way healthcare services are delivered in the United States. Physicians who adapt to team-based care models will be well-positioned to thrive and lead in the midst of an escalating pace of change in the industry.

The power physicians hold today has changed from that of the past, but their role is critical to ensuring improvement in quality, access, and cost of care. No longer will leadership derive from a position of autonomous authority. Rather, physician leadership will depend on physicians' power, knowledge, and skills to influence patient care as part of clinical teams, leadership teams, and governance teams.

The rigors of didactic training and experiential learning positions physicians well for the role of ensuring quality of care for the patients and populations they serve. As clinicians, physicians are uniquely suited to leverage their skills to bolster their position as subject-matter experts in shared clinical decision-making with patients and in health system operations. However, the leadership skills that are crucial for teamwork are not always a part of physician training or culture. They must become so.

Physicians must redesign the profession. This professional redesign requires an introspective understanding of training curricula and how the physician culture should be shaped in the future to improve abilities to lead in patient-centric operations, complex healthcare organizations, and at the national social policy level. The transformation will require continued review of the social and environmental forces that are stressing the physician community and the healthcare system.

Regularly examining the current situation from the perspective of various strategic lenses (e.g., health-centric, economic, political, and social) can uncover changing trends in this complex adaptive system and the changes in communication and relationships that affect the effectiveness of higher quality care and improve patient outcomes in the future. Any passive avoidance as a cultural strategy merely increases strain on the system and contributes to victimization and dysfunctional physician behavior. We need a new way to serve our communities and provide optimal care.

REFERENCES

1. Starr P. *The Social Transformation of American Medicine.* New York, NY: Harper Collins;1982, p. 359.
2. Toffler, A. *Powershift: Knowledge, Wealth, and Violence at the Edge of the 21st Century.* New York: Bantam Books; 1990.
3. Starr, p. 15.
4. McFarland MS, Finks SW, the Medications Right Institute. Medication Optimization: Integration of Comprehensive Medication Management into Practice. *American Health & Drug Benefits*, Am Health Drug Benefits. 2021 Sep; 14(3):11-114.

5. Magee M. The Evolving Patient-Physician Relationship. *Health Politics: Power, Populism and Health.* Bronxville, NY: Spencer Books; 2005, p. 36.

6. Becker's Healthcare. *Consumers vs Patients: Healthcare's Biggest Misunderstanding.* Beacker's Health IT. February 18,, 2015. www.beckershospitalreview.com/healthcare-information-technology/consumers-vs-patients-healthcare-s-biggest-misunderstanding.html.

7. Godolphin W. Shared Decision-making. *Healthc Q.* 2009;12 Spec No Patient: p186-90.

8. Starr, p. 16.

9. Shannon, D. Did You Get an 'A'? *Physician Executive.* Nov/Dec 2007; 33(6):4-8.

10. Campbell EM, Sittig DF, Ash JS, Guappone KP, Dykstra RH. Types of Unintended Consequences Related To Computerized Provider Order Entry. *J Am Med Inform Assoc.* 2006 Sep-Oct;13(5):547-56.

11. Harrison MI, Koppel R, Bar-Lev S. Unintended Consequences of Information Technologies in Health Care--An Interactive Sociotechnical Analysis. *J Am Med Inform Assoc.* 2007 Sep-Oct;14(5):542-9.

12. Koppel R, Wetterneck T, Telles JL, Karsh BT. Workarounds to Barcode Medication Administration Systems: Their Occurrences, Causes, and Threats to Patient Safety. *J Am Med Inform Assoc.* 2008 Jul- Aug;15(4):408-23.

13. Institute of Medicine. Committee on the Robert Wood Johnson Foundation Initiative on the Future of Nursing, at the Institute of Medicine. Summary. In *The Future of Nursing: Leading Change, Advancing Health.* Washington, DC: National Academies Press; 2011, pp. 221-225.

14. Hsiao W. Abnormal Economics in the Health Sector. *Health Policy.* 1995 Apr-Jun;32(1-3):125-39.

15. American Medical Association. Physician-led Team-based Care. American Medical Association. (n.d.). www.ama-assn.org/practice-management/scope-practice/physician-led-team-based-care.

16. American Medical Association. Models of Physician-led Team-based Care. American Medical Association. (n.d.). www.ama-assn.org/sites/ama-assn.org/files/corp/media-browser/public/cms/team-based-models_0.pdf.

17. Freund T, Everett C, Griffiths P, et al.*Skill Mix, Roles and Remuneration in the Primary Care Workforce: Whoe Are the Heatlhcare Professionals in the Primary Care Teams Across The World?* nt J Nurs Stud. 2015 Mar;52(3):727-43. doi: 10.1016/j.ijnurstu.2014.11.014. Epub 2014 Dec 19.

18. Hawklins TP. *2018 Survey of America's Physicians: Practice Patterns and Perspectives.* The Physicians Foundation. 2018. https://physiciansfoundation.org/wp-content/uploads/2018/09/physicians-survey-results-final-2018.pdf.

19. LaPointe J. *Less Than a Third of Docs Owned Independent Pracices in 2018.* Revcycle Intelligence. September 20, 2018. https://revcycleintelligence.com/news/less-than-a-third-of-docs-owned-independent-practices-in-2018.

20. Rubin R. COVID-19's Crushing Effects on Medical Practices, Some of Which Might Not Survive. *JAMA. 2020;324(4):321-323. doi:10.1001/jama.2020.11254.*

21. Frank R, N. T. (2021). Addressing the Risk of Medicare Trust Fund Insolvency. *JAMA. 2021;325(4):341-342. doi:10.1001/jama.2020.26026.*

22. Jacobs P, Rapoport J. Additional Topics in the Demand for Health and Medical Care. In: *The Economics of Health and Medical Care.* 5th ed. Subury, MA: Jones and Bartlett Publishers; 2004. p. 86.

23. Jacobs P, Rapoport J. *The Economics of Health and Medical Care.* 5th ed. Subury, MA: Jones and Bartlett Publishers; 2004. pp. 87-88.

24. Institute of Medicine. Committee on the Robert Wood Johnson Foundation Initiative on the Future of Nursing, at the Institute of Medicine. Summary. In *The Future of Nursing: Leading Change, Advancing Health.* Washington, DC: National Academies Press; 2011. pp. 257-266.

25. United States Government. H.R. 3590, Patient Protection and Affordable Care Act, §5202. Nursing student loan program; §5308. Advanced nursing education grants; §5309. Nurse education, practice and retention grants (2010).

CHAPTER 2: POWERSHIFT AND TEAMBUILDING
Leadership Implications and Health Policy Considerations

Leadership Implications:

1. Recognize the primary importance of the physician-patient relationship and encourage practicing physicians to embrace and cultivate it as a partnership. Reflect upon the physician-patient relationship as critical to the legitimation of professional authority.

2. Foster the development of collaborative relationships with clinical and administrative teammates from multiple professional backgrounds.

Health Policy Considerations:

1. In the development of medical affairs policies at the provider organization level, account for the *workflow* impact of health information technology solutions when defining boundaries, roles, and controls governing physician role.

2. When addressing local and regional health policy reform with community health boards and local governments, understand and communicate the importance of current and prevalent economic and technology trends and their direct impact on the communities being served.

Varieties of Leadership Experience

Power comes from various sources. Leaders' power comes from their ability to influence and organize individuals around a common goal. Societies anoint formal leaders with titles such as king, president, chief executive officer, chief, and manager. Physicians are powerful by virtue of their healing role. Healers are given different titles and have distinct roles, such as physician, shaman, therapist, and priest. The contemporary call for physicians to become better leaders in our healthcare system is therefore intrinsically complex.

Today, effective healthcare leadership requires leaders to develop management, communication, and strategy skills that have historically not been taught in medical school curricula. Although this deficiency is beginning to be addressed in medical education, medical training continues to emphasize clinical competencies rather than the development of leadership skills.[1]

In 2001, Michael S. Woods, MD, wrote an analysis of leadership principles as they apply to healthcare in which he remarked on the dearth of literature on personal leadership development and interpersonal skills in medical education.[2] He observed that leadership of the American healthcare enterprise, once the province of physicians, has become almost exclusively a non-physician activity.[3]

In 2006, the Accreditation Council for Graduate Medical Education issued educational materials under the project title "Educating Physicians for the 21st Century."[4] Their message to facilitators and program directors focused on the six core competencies for physicians in residency that had been identified by the ACGME in 1999. Those six competencies were:

1. Medical knowledge.
2. Patient care.
3. Practice-based learning and improvement.
4. Systems-based practice.

5. Professionalism.

6. Interpersonal and communication skills.

The last three competencies were intended to focus on skills physicians need to strengthen their leadership abilities as they begin their careers. However, even with this emphasis by the ACGME and the strong efforts of those working to educate medical students in didactic training and experiential learning, gaps still exist between what new physicians need to be prepared for leadership and managerial skills necessary to advance in the practice of medicine.

Jerome Groopman, MD, in 2009, argued in his bestselling *How Doctors Think* that physician training creates a particular mindset used in clinical diagnosis that is not conducive to creative thinking. He emphasized the importance of developing non-reductive critical thinking skills to improve clinical diagnosis in ambiguous clinical presentations:

> Clinical algorithms can be useful for run-of-the-mill diagnosis and treatment. . . . But they quickly fall apart when a doctor needs to think outside their boxes, when symptoms are vague, or multiple and confusing, or when test results are inexact. . . . Medicine is, at its core, an uncertain science.[5]

In addition to their importance in the clinical environment when diagnoses are unclear, these creative thinking skills are necessary for influential leadership in the non-clinical environment. Physicians are first educated over several years through didactic methods, followed by a process of experiential learning. This training methodology creates a foundational set of mental processes and analytical abilities that drives the development of clinical reasoning skills.

Similar to Groopman's critique, Woods argues that in order to be effective leaders, "physicians today, and those in training to become physicians, will have to unlearn the sterile, linear reductionist approaches of the past and embrace current personal leadership concepts" that are based on the "softer" skills learned in the social, psychological, organizational, and management sciences.[6]

The inherent competitiveness of physician training does not engender an environment where these crucial creative thinking skills necessary for leadership development are encouraged. According to Woods, the prolonged training necessary to produce technically competent physicians has contributed to a culture in which physicians use technical and intellectual ability as a proxy for leadership.

He believes physicians cling to autonomy over teamwork as a value due to the enormous personal and emotional cost of obtaining their professional credentials, all the while remaining the most risk-averse of all professions not only in terms of patient care but also in terms of openness to trying new business models.

Physician leaders need to collaborate with others to take co-responsibility for costs, resource utilization, quality, patient safety, and the other healthcare macroeconomic problems that are driving healthcare system changes. Physicians need to transition from an overvaluation of professional autonomy to values that encompass more effective leadership traits built on collaborative relationships, systems thinking, and integrated models of care.

These crucial leadership traits can be developed within a variety of leadership frameworks, provided there is a conscious effort to acknowledge their importance and balance the classical clinical reductive training with broader exposure to leadership

THREE THEORIES OF LEADERSHIP

The disciplined study of leadership during the past century can be divided into three phases: the Great Man and Trait phase, the Behavior Phase, and the Situational Phase. Historically, until around 1940, leadership theory attempted to determine the specific traits that make a person an effective leader by studying the "great men" (rarely women) of history. From the 1940s through the 1960s, behavioral theorists dominated, attempting to determine which particular behaviors leaders use to cause others to follow them. From the 1970s through the present day, effective leadership is typically evaluated within the context of the environment in which it occurs.[7]

Consistent with this contemporary emphasis, multiple varieties of physician leadership can be identified within the different environments in which physicians lead. Physicians can lead within the frameworks of situational, transformational, or servant leadership. They can lead in traditional formal leadership roles, but also in innovation, education, physician well-being, research, policy, and in tactical roles in any professional environment in which they reside.

A distinction is often made between leadership and management. "People are led, and resources are managed!" Ledlow and Coppola exclaimed.[8] Management organizes the work of others to improve profitability and increase productivity.

As with other industries, healthcare often uses project management, quality improvement tools, and other methodologies to set and manage the work that must be done to keep an organization running. But there is a moral quality to leadership not necessarily emphasized in such characterizations of management. As Peter Drucker says, "Leadership is doing the right things." At the core, all leadership theory emphasizes a shared set of elements:

- Setting a shared vision for the organization or group.
- Securing and getting the *right* team members and stakeholders on board the ship.
- Motivating the team and stakeholders to work toward the shared vision.
- Building and sharing the strategic plan for achieving the vision.
- Navigating the course for the organization in good and trying times.

Underlying all of these elements is the moral duty to "do the right thing."

In Drucker's framework, leadership is directly tied to ethical obligations. The discourse regarding the moral duty of physicians is typically grounded in the one-to-one physician-patient relationship at the individual level rather than the obligations engendered in an organizational leadership role. The traditional Hippocratic Oath physicians take at medical school graduation "sketches the ethically proper way for physicians to treat their patients."[9] There is no direct acknowledgment of any ethical obligation in a broader leadership context.

The organizational custodianship necessary for leadership in complex healthcare delivery systems requires physicians to re-center their ethical focus on their duties to the individual patient in a larger systems framework in order to provide effective leadership.

John Kotter's classic outline of the duties of a leader includes establishing direction, aligning people, motivating and inspiring, and producing change. If these duties are to have relevance within the physician role, then the physician's ethical obligation to the patient articulated 2,500 years ago by Hippocrates must transcend to the systems level. In that framework, the powers of the traditional healer role (shaman) comingle with the powers of the traditional leader role (chief), and the ethical obligations of the traditional physician role rise to a powerful multi-dimensional integrated model that will drive the health system to a patient-centered, high-value model.

The critical linkage in both the individual physician-to-patient role and the physician leadership role is the relationship and moral duty to people. Leadership's role of inspiring, motivating, and enabling change only comes about through the leader's relationship with people. Resources are managed, but people are led.

Drucker, Kouzes and Posner, Blake and Mouton, McGregor, and Stogdill and Coon all emphasized in their work on management and leadership theory the importance of interpersonal relationships. Their business literature translators such as Peter Senge, Ken Blanchard, Jim Collins, and John Kotter interpreted their work at the organizational level and added insights into leadership effectiveness pertinent to the business culture.

For example, in *Good to Great* and *Built to Last,* Collins asserts the necessity of having a "core ideology" for lasting business success:

> Instilling core values (essential and enduring tenets) and core purpose (fundamental reason for being beyond just making money) as principles to guide decisions and inspire people throughout the organization over an extended period of time.[10]

For physician leaders, the core ideology encapsulated in the Hippocratic Oath can be integrated into the mission, vision, and values of the organizations to which they are responsible, just as it serves as the basis for ethical patient care. Ethical leadership that encompasses these physician-centric principles can be identified in three key approaches: situational, transformational, and servant leadership (Table 1).[11]

Situational Leadership

Chaudry *et al.* use the concept of situational leadership to characterize physician leadership traits required for change management. They affirm the necessity of recognizing the need for change and focus on four roles that can be assumed to affect this change: the coach, the delegator, the supporter, or the traditional leader.[12] Within this framework, the importance of trust in one's team is crucial.

In their clinical work environment, physicians play leadership roles within the situational leadership framework every day. The well-choreographed team in the operating theater is the classic example of the traditional physician leadership role in the situational context, where the surgeon, the anesthesiologist, and all the other members of the healthcare team work together in very prescribed roles to deliver safe and effective clinical outcomes.

In the expanded situational leadership roles necessary in the 21st-century healthcare environment, physicians must also learn to lead such complex teams in process improvement, such as the adoption of such patient safety

Table 1.

Leadership Styles		
SITUATIONAL	**TRANSFORMATIONAL**	**SERVANT**
Is adaptable to specific situations	Influences subordinates to drive forward "ethically inspired goals transcending self-interest"	Engages in active listening
Assumes one of four roles: coaching, supporting, delegating, or leading		Demonstrates empathy for workers and peers
	Four central components:	
Understands need for workers' empowerment and recognition	1. Idealized influence 2. Inspirational motivation 3. Intellectual stimulations 4. Individualized consideration	Is a strong communicator of concepts
Knows his or her strengths but adjusts when needed		Possesses strong persuasive abilities
		Exerts a healing influence on individuals and institutions
	Facilitates team growth through individualized mentoring or coaching relationships	Establishes a community in the workplace
Recognizes the need for change		

measures as checklists, patient signoffs on correct-side surgery, and protocol-driven infection control processes.[13] The expertise of other team members must be supported and encouraged without diminishing the traditional clinical roles of physicians.

Transformational Leadership

The transformational leadership model of Xirasanger *et al.* approaches physician leadership from the perspective of influencing others to "ethically inspired goals that transcend self-interest."[14] In the clinic, physicians must influence patients to make healthy lifestyle changes, including smoking cessation, appropriate diet and exercise, and medication adherence.

The "good doctor" is often perceived as one who has a good rapport with patients. While not emphasized in medical training, a good bedside manner is nonetheless what patients value in their physicians, as they take clinical competency as a given. As transformative leaders in our healthcare delivery system, physicians must translate the "bedside manner" to the organizational level, facilitating team growth by mentoring and inspiring. By focusing on the mission and values of the healthcare organization and modeling their behavior accordingly, physicians become better leaders.

Servant Leadership

A third conceptual framework for evaluating leadership is the servant leadership model.[15] Although a number of management thought leaders have written about servant leadership, two of them are particularly pertinent to physician leadership. First is Robert Greenleaf, who believed:

> The first and most important choice a leader makes is the choice to serve, without which, one's capacity to lead is profoundly limited.[16]

Servant leadership is applicable in professional roles in spiritual/religious organizations, academic, government, and healthcare sectors, where service to others is intrinsic to the organization purpose and focus.

Joseph Jaworski, the founder of the American Leadership Forum, is the author of *Synchronicity: The Path of Inner Leadership*. His work focuses on servant leadership as deriving from one's inner values. Jaworski explains that the essence of the servant leader starts with a commitment to listen to the inner voice and allow one to participate in the unfolding of the generative order[17] that can lead to predictable miracles. He concludes that:

> The leadership that can bring forth predictable miracles is more about being than doing. It is about our orientation of character, our state of inner activity.[18]

Ten characteristics best describe servant leadership[19]:

1. Building community
2. Awareness
3. Persuasion
4. Conceptualization
5. Foresight
6. Stewardship
7. Empathy
8. Listening
9. Commitment to growth of people
10. Healing

Just as the characteristics of empathy, listening, and commitment to growth of people are necessary for the development of the healer role for physicians, these 10 traits build on one another in the essential development of physician leaders.

In the uncertainty of the current healthcare climate, providers of healthcare are anxious. Income instability, loss of autonomy, increasingly competitive markets, loss of status, changes in payment models, and insufferable technology have created an environment of low morale among physicians in many healthcare organizations. However, within the servant leader role, physicians can refocus on their strengths, which underlie the healing role inherent in servant leadership. In a new role as healers of the healthcare delivery system, physicians can be reinvigorated with a focus on the values inherent in their traditional servant role as healers of patients.

GOOD PHYSICIAN LEADERSHIP REQUIRES AN UNDERSTANDING OF GOVERNANCE

Critical for today's physicians is greater insight into organizational governance as a cultural requirement for leadership. The anticipated shift toward a more value-driven healthcare system is driving clinical integration strategies, healthcare system consolidations and realignments, and the emergence of new models of healthcare delivery such as accountable care organizations, patient-centered medical homes, virtual primary care, and nationally scaled physician practice organizations. Having physicians in leadership positions in these new organizations will be crucial to their success.[20]

However, many otherwise excellent potential physician leaders have not had experience in leadership roles with governance structures other than medical staffs or physician practices. Consequently, healthcare organizations valuing physician leadership seek organizations with historical success developing physician leaders and incorporating them into governance structure.

Physicians traditionally trained in command-and-control environments as "heroic lone healers" may be seen as "collaboratively challenged" such that "medical training on the whole conspires against great leadership."[21] Nonetheless, substantial data show that institutions that are physician-led perform at higher level than those that are manager-led in quality and patient safety.

The Mayo Clinic is one such organization that has been studied both in the healthcare industry and as a business model relevant in other industries.[22] A 2009 Commonwealth Fund case study on the Mayo Clinic addressed the issue of physician engagement in leadership:

> The organization is physician-led at all levels and operates through physician committees and a shared governance philosophy in which physician leaders work with administrative partners in a horizontal, consensus-driven structure.[23]

Physicians at the Mayo Clinic serve in rotations through various committees, and its Board of Governors is composed primarily of physician leaders. Year after year, Mayo ranks among the world's best healthcare institutions.

In 2021, it maintained its ranking as the number one hospital in the world by the BBC while maintaining its rank at the top (or near the top) U.S. hospital with *U.S. News and World Report*s for 27 years.

It is not coincidental that organizations that incorporate physicians into their governance structure, such as the Carilion Clinic, Geisinger Health System, the Cleveland Clinic, and the Mayo Clinic, are identified as operational models for healthcare delivery system innovation, as these organizations have excelled and set benchmarks for physician leadership in the industry. In fact, although only 235 of 6,500 hospitals in the United States have physicians as chief executive officers, research demonstrates that hospital quality scores are on average 25% higher when the CEO is a physician.[24]

There are tremendous pressures on healthcare organizations to continuously improve quality and safety while lowering costs in an economically constrained environment. Thus, physician leaders must address not only the need for clinical excellence but also administration and support operations through the integration of multidisciplinary groups and individuals while addressing the challenge of how to maintain a highly motivated and engaged workforce.[25]

Applying change management principles is essential to addressing these challenges. Leaders involved in governance committees/boards also face the challenges of:

- Balancing competing interests for health system resources and priorities.
- Determining appropriate affiliations and alliances in a competitive, consolidating business environment.
- Adhering to benchmarks for evaluating best practices within the context of the organization's mission.
- Practicing fiduciary oversight of financial resources, including meeting capital requirements, bond covenants, and cash flow needs.

These issues are not traditionally encountered in the course of a physician's medical education; so, developing an understanding of strategies and tactics for handling the issues collaboratively is essential for physician leaders.

As physician leadership becomes increasingly important at the administrative and board levels of healthcare organizations, their contribution must be appropriate to the structures and essential duties of these governing bodies.

Boards of trustees have three essential legal duties: the duty of obedience, the duty of care, and the duty of loyalty. Within the duty of obedience, a board is accountable to its community (in the case of nonprofit organizations) or to its shareholders (in the case of for-profit organizations) and holds the organization's assets in trust for that community or those shareholders. Each board member has equal responsibilities and obligations, and as a body, the board should be externally focused rather than inwardly focused on operations, which is essentially the responsibility of the administration.

In the duty of care, the board sets policy and direction on which the administration acts. In the duty of loyalty, board members must set the interests of the organization above self-interest.

Physicians who are part of a healthcare organization board must understand the distinction between their duties as board members in contradistinction to their duties as physicians. A board has collective authority. Physicians, who are used to authority as individuals in the professional role, must take care not to speak from a voice of individual authority rather than as a member of a collective whole.

Likewise, the physician's experience as a clinician within a healthcare organization can lead to the temptation to misperceive the board governance role as one that is inwardly focused on administrative and operational aspects of the organization. Finally, the potential conflicts of interest that naturally exist between a physician on the board of an organization in which they might have staff privileges or ownership interest must be transparent and openly acknowledged. Adequate orientation for physicians participating in organizational governance is therefore essential in creating maximum benefit for healthcare organizations that are bringing physician input into the boardroom.

As physicians are increasingly needed in health system management and administrative roles, their grounding in the frontline perspective of direct patient care experience can contribute to critical improvements in operational aspects, particularly in areas concerned with patient safety and quality of care. However, the one-to-one relationship of patient care has a very different function than administrative work, which often requires collaborating with the committee members, working with teams of employees, and making resource management decisions that are foreign to many physicians' training and experience.

Physician input into policy analyses and decision-making that affect care processes is essential for organizational success moving forward, so exposure to management as an academic discipline will be increasingly important for physicians participating in leadership in healthcare organizations.

EFFECTIVE HEALTHCARE ORGANIZATIONS REQUIRE COLLABORATIVE CLINICAL LEADERSHIP

As technology advancements have enhanced our abilities to tear down silos and to increase levels of synergistic work, interdisciplinary cross-functional teaming efforts between various healthcare professionals have emerged and become more commonplace, resulting in high-performing work practices.[26] The collaborative clinical leadership model can provide physician leaders and others in matrix organizations with a structural model to help mitigate governance-level challenges inherent in the current complex healthcare delivery system.

Physician leaders must develop strong collaboration skills to guide their organizations through the myriad transformational issues that continue to affect the healthcare delivery system. Effective collaborative clinical leadership is built on four fundamental elements:

1. Foundational components for an effective healthcare organization.
2. Change imperatives for successfully meeting current industry shortcomings.
3. Teamwork transactions for effectively working in an organization.
4. Accountability to individual patients and community in an organization's mission, vision, and values.

Organizational change is unavoidable within the shifting models of care delivery and ongoing national policy reforms. Collaborative clinical leadership provides a structure within which mission-oriented goals focused on improving the quality of patient care and reducing unnecessary growth in healthcare expenditures can be organized.[27]

Foundations. Establishing a solid foundation for the collaborative clinical leadership model is crucial to overcoming challenges and achieving stability through change.

Five essential elements create the core foundation for the model: a future-focused *vision* of improvement, *values* incorporating the IOM's six aims, re-emphasis on patient-centric models as the *ethical* component of patient care, a *scientific* focus on evidence, and care that is *engineered* to be high performing and reliable (Table 2).

Imperatives. Effective health organizations must perform three essential activities in order to meet the challenges of paradigm-shifting changes occurring in the industry. *Cross-functional teaming* becomes normative as levels of integration across disciplines increase over time. *Population health*

Table 2.

	Foundation for Collaborative Clinical Leadership Model
Vision	A foundational direction for the organization linked to a future state defined by improvement and achievement.
Values	Standards and beliefs that guide an organization with a focus on the Institute of Medicine's Six Aims or other goal directed principles.
Science	Focus on evidence-based practices and standards with application in decision-making.
Engineering	Application of a methodological approach to the design, initiation, or redesigns of care processes that ensure optimal performance and reliability.
Ethical	Strong emphasis on patient-centeredness as the key ethical element of the foundation.

improvement becomes a strategic activity with the shift toward value-based payment models.

Finally, comprehensive and effective *communication* strategies are developed. Inadequate communication can lead to decreased efficiency, poor quality patient care, and decreased capacity to reduce healthcare expenditures.

Teamwork. Gittel *et al.* recognized that high-performing work systems depend on cross-functional work practices in which leaders from each of the disciplines are capable of efficiently collaborating.[28] Achieving transformative change in healthcare requires the formation of new work relationships and the elimination of barriers and silos inherent in current work structures.

A commitment to achieving operational integration of services to enhance and improve the healthcare services for patients must be a common priority of all the professional disciplines that make up the current healthcare workforce.

Accountability. Starting at the top of organizational hierarchies and penetrating throughout the organization, leaders must embrace full responsibility for delivering effective patient care services.

Traditionally, physicians have been held accountable through professional standards, medical staff bylaws, licensure, and the tort system in which physicians are responsible for clinical decisions in ways that are distinctly different from other healthcare professionals. But physicians have not necessarily been held accountable for organizational goals nor for the overall cost or quality of care.

Officers of healthcare organizations traditionally have been held accountable for organizational financial performance and meeting accreditation standards. Still, they typically have been shielded from personal liability for organizational performance unless they have committed criminally negligent acts.

Recent regulatory changes in HIPAA Privacy and Security, however, can lead to personal fines as well as financial penalties for organization leaders, and value-based payment models create performance incentives that require integrated responsibility.

QUANTITATIVE SKILLS ARE CRUCIAL ASSETS FOR PHYSICIAN LEADERS

Traditional medical training teaches quantitative analyses within the context of clinical diagnosis, but physician leaders must generalize their quantitative skills to be broadly applicable in performance management.

Pay-for-performance components of value-based contracts, population-based payments, and payments based on clinically measurable outcomes continue to drive the need for clinical leadership adept at quantitative analysis at the health systems level. Patient care outcomes, clinical benchmarking, adherence to best practices and evidence-based medicine standards, transparency of patient satisfaction, and financial performance require clinical leaders who are comfortable with quantitative analyses as a competitive asset.

Performance Reporting at the Individual Clinician Level. The days of limited transparency of quality among physician peers and healthcare provider organizations are over. With the passage of MACRA legislation in 2015, all federally funded professional payments became tied to performance through MIPS and Advanced Alternative Payment models. Quality reporting is now a federal policy with financially differentiated payments for services embedded in the law. The healthcare industry now competes based on meeting quality and cost benchmarks rather than on volume of services or the non-quantitative reputation of the provider.

Performance Reporting at the Organizational Level. To effectively manage, healthcare organizations require quantitative performance benchmarking using executive dashboards and other clinical, financial, and operational benchmarking and reporting tools. Physician leadership in the selection, monitoring, and evaluation of key clinical performance indicators is crucial.

As members of boards of directors, medical executive committees, or other governance structures, physician leaders also need skills in the language of business analysis to provide the appropriate fiduciary oversight and performance management needed by officers and management of their healthcare organizations.

Ongoing healthcare payment reform will accelerate the need for the financially constrained industry to address critical areas of performance. Quality and safety, physician satisfaction, patient satisfaction, revenue cycle management, and operational efficiency and effectiveness will become integrated indicators of organizational performance.

Performance Assessment Using the Donabedian Framework. Driving organizations to achieve better health outcomes is one of the essential functions for physician leaders, and some research indicates physician-led health systems have higher average quality ratings than non-physician-led systems.[29] Increasingly sophisticated assessments of health outcomes performance will be transparently reported for integrated delivery systems, retail-based healthcare organizations, independent physician practices, and individual physicians.

Physician leaders should bring their clinical expertise to the boardroom in those organizations able to perform at the highest level and impact the health outcomes of the communities they serve. Providing insights into the meaning of outcome measurements and their relation to the critical areas to measure the "health of the organization" should be part of the inherent mission in measuring and evaluating progress.

In 1966, Avedis Donabedian proposed his quality framework[30] as a methodology for evaluating the quality of medical care. He proposed that the quality of medical care is affected at three levels: (1) structures of care, (2) processes of care, and (3) health outcomes. Donabedian's application remains a relevant assessment tool from which many quality reporting initiatives, executive dashboards, and other performance reports can be evaluated.

Assessing the structures of care may entail evaluating the facilities, finances, and effectiveness of capital equipment and technologies for use in the organization. Processes of care may involve analysis of the efficiencies of clinical workflows across clinical disciplines. Understanding the degree of integration that exists from technologies and shared clinician resources is important for physician executives to evaluate operational and administrative processes.

The performance assessment framework built on structure, processes, and outcomes of care developed by Donabedian can serve as pillars to support physician leaders within the wide variety of leadership experiences in which they work.

REFERENCES

1. Hollomon D, Campion B. Physicians, Leading, and Dialogue. *Group Practice Journal.* June 2007; 20-23.

2. Woods M. *Applying Personal Leadership Principles to Health Care: The DEPO Principle.* Tampa, FL: American College of Physician Executives; 2001, p. 3.

3. Woods, p. 14.

4. Accreditation Council for Graduate Medical Education. ACGME Outcome Project: Educating Physicians for the 21st Century. www.acgme.org/outcome/e-learn/e_powerpoint.asp.

5. Groopman J. *How Doctors Think.* New York, NY: Houghton Mifflin Company; 2007, pp. 5-7.

6. Woods, p. 66.

7. Ledlow G, Coppola N. *Leadership for Health Professionals: Theory, Skills, and Applications.* Sudbury, MA: Jones and Bartlett Learning; 2011, pp. 10-11.

8. Ledlow G, Coppola N., p. 1.

9. Loewy E. Oaths for Physicians – Necessary Protection or Elaborate Hoax? *MedGenMed.* 2007; 9(1):7.

10. Collins J. *Good to Great.* New York, NY: HarperCollins Publishers, Inc. ; 2001, p. 198.

11. Flareau B, Bohn J, Konschak C. *Accountable Care Organizations: A Roadmap for Success.* Virginia Beach, VA: Convergent Publishing; 2011, p. 51.

12. Chaudry J, Jain A, McKenzie S, Schwartz RW. Physician Leadership: The Competencies of Change. *J. Surg Educ.* 2008;65(3):213-220.

13. Gawande A. Chapter 2. The Checklist. *In: The Checklist Manifesto. How To Get Things Right.* New York, NY: Metropolitan Books; 2009, pp. 35-47.

14. Xirasagar S, Samuels ME, Curtain TF. (February 2006). Management Training of Physician Executives, Their Leadership Style, and Care Management Performance: An Empirical study. *Am J Manag Care.* 2006;12(2):101-108.

15. Schwartz RW, Tumblin TF. The Power of Servant Leadership To Transform Health Care Organizations for the 21st-Centruy Economy. *Arch Surg.* 2002;137(12):1419-1427.

16. Jaworski J. Introduction. *Synchronicity: The Inner Path of Leadership.* San Francisco, CA: Berrett-Koehler Publishers;1996, p. 1.

17. Pratt D. David Bohm and the Implicate Order. *Sunrise Magazine.* February/March 1993.

18. Jaworski, Chapter 24: Creating the Future. In: *Synchronicity,* p. 185.

19. Joseph E, Winston B. A Correlation of Servant Leadership, Leader Trust, and Organizational Trust. *Leadership & Organization Development Journal.* 2005;26(1);6-22.

20. Flareau, p. 13; Fisher ES, McClellan MB, Bertko J, et al. Fostering Accountable Health Care: Moving Forward in Medicare. *Health Aff (Millwood)* 2009;28(2):w219-w231.

21. Stoller, JK, Goodall A, Baker A. Why the Best Hospitals are Managed by Doctors. *Harvard Business Review*. December 27, 2016. https://hbr.org/2016/12/why-the-best-hospitals-are-managed-by-doctors.

22. Berry LL, Seltman KD. *Management Lessons From Mayo Clinic: Inside One of the World's Most Admired Service Organizations*. New York, NY: McGraw-Hill; 2008.

23. McCarthy D, Mueller K, Wrenn J. Mayo Clinic: Multidisciplinary Teamwork, Physician-led Governance, and Patient-Centered Culture Drive World-class Health Care. *Commonwealth Fund*. Aug 2009; (27)1306.

24. Goodall AH. Physician-leaders and hospital performance: Is there an association? *Soc Sci Med*. July 2011. Discussion Paper No 5830. www. science/article/pii/S0277953611003819; Gunderman R, Kanter SL. Perspective: Educating Physicians to Lead Hospitals. *Academic Medicine*. 2009; (84)10;1348-1351.

25. Stock D, Bentley J. Building and Keeping a Thriving Workforce: The Board's Role. *Trustee*. 2009; Jan;62(1):31-2.

26. Gittell J, Seidner R, Wimbush J. A Relational Model of How High-Performance Work Systems Work.
Organization Science. 2010;21(2):490-506; Flareau, p. 61.

27. Center for Medicare & Medicaid Services. CMS-1345-P. Medicare Program; Medicare Shared Savings Program: Accountable Care Organizations. Proposed Rule. March 31, 2011. pp. 13-14.

28. Gittell J, Seidner R, Wimbush J. A Relational Model of How High-Performance Work Systems Work. *Organization Science*. 2010;21(2):490-506.

29. Tasi, MC, Keswani A, Bozic KJ, Does Physician Leadership Affect Hospital Quality, Operational Efficiency, and Financial Performance? *Health Care Manage Rev*. Jul/Sep 2019;44(3):256-262.doi:10.1097/HMR.0000000000000173.

30. Donabedian A. Evaluating the Quality of Medical Care. *Milbank Quarterly* 2005;83(4):691-729. Reprinted from *Milbank Memorial Fund Quarterly* 1966;44(3):166–203.

CHAPTER 3: VARIETIES OF LEADERSHIP EXPERIENCE

Leadership Implications and Health Policy Considerations

Leadership Implications:

1. Evaluate how the different leadership theories might frame your own leadership qualities through different lenses.
2. Learn how your organization is governed and evaluate how that impacts the scope of your leadership opportunities.
3. Investigate the scope of collaborative clinical leadership in your organization.

Health Policy Considerations:

1. Develop performance management processes at the organizational, community, or governmental level.
2. Support or ensure organizational participation in requests for input on legislative actions.
3. Evaluate need for action on legislative reforms with constituents and define your organization's role.

Barriers to Healthy Change

The time has come for radical change . . . The management of medical care has become too important to leave to doctors, who, after all, are not managers to begin with.[1]

Fortune Magazine, Jan. 1970

The medical-industrial complex has segregated the roles of physician clinician and organizational manager for a generation, all the while decrying the lack of physicians with adequate leadership skills (Figure 1). The labyrinthine structures of health systems and multiple payers have been built on organizations designed for pre-Information Age industrial systems. These organizations are designed for the high-volume output of products and operate under the assumptions of a fee-for-service business model.

As the complexity of the healthcare system accelerated with technological advances and financial optimization, the skills required of a physician in, for example, the cardiac catheter lab, diverged markedly from the skills necessary to supervise and manage the resources of large, capital-intense, complex medical facilities and institutions. During the past 50 years, the solo practitioner in a small office whose spouse "did the books" became increasingly obsolete, as the processes necessary to operate in a complex regulatory and managed-care environment progressively become over-burdensome.

Whereas most physicians operated their practices as small, independent businesses in the past, the majority of today's physicians are employees of large, complex organizations in which they are expected to be highly productive frontline service workers.

Currently, fewer physicians own their own practices than are employed by hospitals, and nearly 70% of physicians under age 40 were employees in 2018.[2] Unfortunately, employed physicians have higher rates of burnout than independent physicians, with loss of control over their lives often cited as a reason.[3]

The pigeonholing of physicians into clinical productivity roles has led to a dearth of management expertise in the profession and pigeonholing of

The Classic Description of the Physician Leadership Dual Roles	
Physician	**Manager**
Autonomous, makes decisions alone	Uses teamwork, probably involved in line reporting
Works one-on-one	Works primarily in groups
Empathetic	Objective
Crisis-oriented	Long-range planner
Quality-oriented	Cost-oriented
Enjoys immediate tangible results	Must often delay gratification and enjoy process
Accustomed to controlled chaos	Planned schedule, more inherent flexibility
Sees people as materials/objects	Sees people as resources to be managed
Is a doer	Is a delegator, gets things done through others
Reacts	Proacts
Is authoritarian in practice style	Delegates authority
Specialist orientation	Generalist orientation
Discipline oriented	Socially oriented

Figure 1.

leadership opportunities. The traditional distinction between physician and manager has been studied by those seeking to understand the "dilemma of the dual role" in physician executive education and draws a stark contrast between the two roles.[4]

Physician leadership will be increasingly needed in the emerging redesigned healthcare system. Both the traditional physician clinical role and the traditional business manager role will need to adapt to new circumstances. More integrated roles will emerge that do not starkly bifurcate the clinical and management roles. Value-based care payment arrangements, nontraditional entrants into the healthcare industry such as Amazon, and ongoing accelerated technology adoption will require a post-industrial leadership model that requires more integrated skills and roles for success.

Understanding the leadership barriers that physicians throughout the healthcare industry face will help reset a successful professional course for the future. Failure to address these barriers may adversely affect the capacity to improve the quality, access, and affordability of healthcare. Therefore, this discussion centers on several types of organizational barriers physician leaders face across many healthcare settings.

STRUCTURAL BARRIERS

The IOM's *Crossing the Quality Chasm* identified four underlying reasons for inadequate quality of care across the U.S. health system: (1) the growing complexity of science and technology, (2) an increase in chronic conditions, (3) a poorly organized delivery system, and (4) constraints on exploiting the revolution in information technology.[5]

The U.S. healthcare system is one of the most complex industries in the world. Inadequately designed and applied systems of care in the fragmented, fee-for-service, episodically focused U.S. healthcare delivery system often fail to provide appropriate services, instead delivering services that are neither effective, efficient, equitable, timely, patient-centered, nor safe. However, physician leaders may be the source of innovative solutions within this complex environment.

Physician engagement and involvement in research application and policy development that takes place in academic, commercial, and governmental research and development settings may create the opportunity to improve clinical outcomes in a more cost-effective way if physicians are active at both researcher and leadership levels. A professional focus on the role of science in developing new interventions and medical technologies that transition from the bench to the bedside to improve the delivery of high-quality care is a space within the industry in which physician leaders may have a significant impact.

Inherent barriers to progress occur within the domain of scientific research, such as ownership of intellectual property rights. Industry competition poses challenges regarding disclosure of discoveries along with rights to future revenue streams and royalties from the commercialization of new drug therapies and medical technologies due to the dependency of contemporary scientific research on high levels of capitalization. In this era of declining reimbursement and constant emphasis on delivering higher quality care at lower cost, having physician leaders who can navigate these challenges and create the pathways that drive the capital markets toward technological innovations that deliver value is essential to achieving scientific research objectives that improve the quality and cost of care.

The delay in widespread clinical adoption of the most up-to-date medical research has been estimated to be as much as 15 years and is accelerating with the exponential increase in medical knowledge. The lag in going from bench research to bedside application is a barrier to the widespread adoption of evidence-based medicine guidelines that improve clinical outcomes.

While rapid advancement of health information technologies and knowledge management applications over the past four decades has accelerated and expanded physicians' abilities to search for and identify best available clinical evidence, scant financial resources have been put into comparative effectiveness research and analyses on alternative medical interventions, treatments, and care delivery processes. Point-of-service, evidence-based best practice information would decrease the overall cost of care by eliminating unnecessary, potentially harmful, or wasteful care.

The IOM's Roundtable on Evidence-Based Medicine in 2008 identified the need for financial investment in best practices research, prompting federal funding to the tune of a billion dollars for multi-year studies for comparative effectiveness research. In, 2010 the Patient Protection and Affordable Care Act established the Patient-Centered Outcomes Research Trust Fund to finance research that can help patients make better-informed decisions about their healthcare choices. In 2019, Congress amended the authorizing law to receive ongoing revenue from statutory appropriations and a few assessed on private insurance and self-insured health plans.

The emphasis on comparative effectiveness will require physician leadership in setting clinical guidelines and policies. Barriers to the development of more widespread evidence-based medicine practice patterns must be addressed with physician leaders working with payers to navigate between standardization of care processes and disruptive innovations that may or may not improve care.

The current healthcare system can be characterized as a *complex adaptive system* that is fragmented and decentralized.[6] Whereas physician leaders recognize the need for reengineering the healthcare system, the fragmentation and decentralization have led to several problems for tertiary care hospitals, physician practices, and other care providers in delivering adequate access and coordination of care.

Initiatives such as patient-centered medical homes, clinical integration programs, accountable care organizations, retail-based clinics, and virtual care platforms intended to transform care delivery face the challenges inherent in all complex adaptive systems: the need to manage unanticipated outcomes that result from changes to the system.

New models of care are diffusing throughout the industry during a time when traditional medical practices and hospital organizations are being stressed by workforce shortages, new regulatory requirements, new technologies, decreased reimbursements from private and public payers, merging of cultures brought on by the industry consolidation necessary for clinical integration, new competitors in the industry such as Amazon and retail pharmacies, and the global pandemic.

The ongoing industry innovation is taking place within the context of chang-ing healthcare population needs. The rise in importance of chronic disease management is the positive outcome of ongoing medical advances in treat-ing heart disease, cancer, and metabolic disorders. As individuals survive previously fatal cancers and have statins and stents to reduce morbidity and mortality from acute cardiovascular disease, the population is growing older and living with a larger number of chronic diseases.

As the number of chronic diseases per patient increases, the associated cost of medical care accelerates. On a per-capita basis, the annual cost of care for a Medicare patient with no chronic conditions is less than $1,000 annually; that cost rises with the number of conditions such that those who have more than five chronic conditions cost Medicare in excess of $17,000 annually — more than twice the average.[7]

The CDC's national campaigns for Healthy People 2010, 2020, and 2030 establish objectives focused on reducing the prevalence of diabetes, cancer, osteoporosis, arthritis, and other chronic conditions. The 355 core objec-tives of Healthy People 2030 set data-driven national objectives to improve health and wellbeing over the next decade based on an effort to affect the costs associated with these chronic diseases through population awareness and lifestyle change.[8]

Physician leaders will need to focus additional resources on chronic disease management in order to improve the population's overall health. Strong phy-sician leadership is required at the community level to eliminate barriers to the reduction in the prevalence of these conditions. Changing lifestyle habits of the population is not the traditional realm of one-on-one doctor-patient communication, so meaningful transformation of the physician role to one that encompasses population health management is necessary.

One final barrier noted by the IOM was constraints on exploiting the revolution in information technology. The tremendous growth in consumer access to health and medical information has occurred during the past two decades, often bypassing the traditional physician role of providing medical information. Traditional remuneration is based on face-to-face office visits, which is not necessarily the most pertinent interaction necessary for good medical care in a world of e-mail, Twitter, Facebook, TikTok, and other social media platforms.

While consumers as a whole are becoming more educated with the vast amount of health information available through the web, the lack of under-lying medical framework can leave them with only a partial understanding of disease/condition symptoms and risks/benefits from various medical interventions and treatments along with side effects or potential unintended adverse consequences.

Online anti-science influencers such as anti-Vaxers have been enormously challenging to address, as media influencers often disseminate invalid information at a rate that cannot be tackled with traditional one-on-one doctor-patient interactions. Traditional methods of providing clinical information are increasingly inadequate. Physicians are challenged by the need to track the occurrence and effectiveness of alternative patient communication, to have 24/7 availability, to incorporate remote monitoring information, and to be able to incorporate and act on patient-derived data.

The transition to a value- and quality-driven healthcare system away from the volume- and transaction-based system requires a redesign of physician-patient communication tools and associated financial reimbursement for use such that both the provider side of the industry and the payer side (as led by CMS) are able to implement more value-oriented programs that improve accountability, accessibility, transparency, and improved resource utilization.

PSYCHOSOCIAL BARRIERS

The ramifications of not addressing psychosocial aspects of the physician role are not only barriers to physician leadership, but also have an enormous impact on physicians' personal wellbeing, their families, their patients, and the organizations and the communities in which they practice. How physicians view and interpret actions and situations affects their intuitive analysis of situations and their clinical decision-making and managerial judgment for their healthcare organizations.

Status Anxiety. While the impact of the pandemic has increased interest in medical school,[9] the medical profession's traditional high social status continues to be challenged by numerous circumstances, including those inherent in the changing cultural landscape, such as:

- The American public's increasing frustration with potential financial conflicts of interest inherent for physicians in both fee-for-service and managed-care capitation payment systems.
- The increasing egalitarian nature of American culture.
- The loss of monopoly power over medical knowledge, which is accelerated by the Internet.
- The fragmentation of the profession brought on by the necessity of specialization in technologically advanced healthcare delivery.

Although American physicians have some of the highest incomes in the world, the profession's control over these incomes continues to erode, one specialty at a time. Payers cut physician fees in an effort to combat the costly effect of accelerated use of healthcare, and health systems base compensation on RVU productivity standards and push compensation to the mean to demonstrate fair market value and avoid regulatory scrutiny. Consequently, physicians find themselves working harder, seeing more patients, and performing more administrative tasks in order to maximize their earnings.

Many physicians believe it wasn't supposed to be this way. Traditionally, physicians were selected for medical school based on competitive characteristics, as described here:

> After a grueling four-year undergraduate curriculum of science course, the ones with the highest grade point averages are selected for entry into medical school. That grueling four-year curriculum includes demonstrating the ability to memorize huge amounts of material and produce memorized knowledge readily (a trait unlikely to encourage use of reference works). The competition with other pre-med students for the top grade point average tends to produce a non-collaborative, non-team oriented, self-centered individual (or select for those who are), because the ones who help others only decrease the amount by which they are or can be seen as "out of the ordinary.[10]

Thus, the need for physicians to work within a collaborative, team-based work environment may be constrained by those traits that make for successful medical school selection. From medical school matriculation through the next 7-12 years, the physician is trained to work in one-on-one situations where they are the dominant authority.[11]

The evolving demands for more accountability for the fragmented healthcare system is not conducive to the *status quo* values of:

> . . . independence of providers, simple structure, professional norms, and collegial relationships in which most physicians were trained and acculturated. Accountability is a direct challenge to physician sovereignty and autonomy and pushes the need for cultural refining of the medical profession.[12]

But for physicians who spend 11-16 years of their life in professional training adaptive for one cultural circumstance, the psychosocial impact of this change can be enormously stressful. Moreover, with the average student debt at graduation now reaching $215,900,[13] their ability to change their life course mid-stream and adapt to reduced economic circumstances and new behaviors is further strained by expectations of payoffs for risks and tradeoffs made much earlier in life. The impact of medical education and acculturation on physician capacity for effective leadership must be addressed.

Perfectionism. Engrained in many physicians through inherent characteristics and the medical education process is the drive always to make the correct diagnosis. Whether the issue they are addressing is about patient care, organizational personnel, technology selection, or partnership formation issues, their drive to make perfect decisions can cause significant stress and directly impact physicians throughout their careers.

Situational Trauma. Medical education can in and of itself be traumatic. But the traumatic impact of physicians' role as authority decision-makers can be intense. Unlike most other members of the healthcare team, physicians are still sued as individuals in malpractice cases. The legal system still views the physician role as one of individual responsibility in the team environment. The day-to-day patient care responsibilities in serious conditions — death, surgeries, emotion crises — are intrinsic in the physician role, but as human beings, physicians must manage the accompanying stress like anyone else.

The toll that stress takes on the physician community is cloaked in a culture that does not encourage forthright communication about physician distress. During the pandemic, physician stress has been at an all-time high, with anxiety over a second surge, crisis fatigue, and workplace safety eroding resiliency.[14] Two-thirds of physicians in the United States report worsening levels of burnout and loneliness during the COVID-19 pandemic, with 43% reporting it has put stress on their relationships and 62% reporting up to a 50% reduction in income.[15]

Beliefs. Feelings that certain tenets and principles are true based on cultural and societal norms shape a physician's understanding of what is ethical. The medical education system must mitigate the impact that differing beliefs have on a physician's ability to treat patients and collaborate with colleagues from diverse backgrounds. However, each individual's personal beliefs may inherently lead to barriers for progress in patient care or practice and organization management.

Limit/Boundary Establishment. Physicians must be able to establish boundaries in patient-physician relations as well as collegial relations within the broader context of the organizations they work in and in their community.

Relational Influence. Traditional male physician and female nurse roles of authoritative command, with a passive-aggressive response, can no longer be presumed normative in environments that rely on teamwork for safe delivery of patient care. However, ongoing cultural gender expectations may continue to influence patient care and personal interaction.

Interactions between female doctors and nurses may be challenged by the Western cultural tendency to equalize relationships within the gender. This cultural expectation to push for horizontal relationships between women may lead to ambiguity in situations where a clear line of authority in the medical decision-making process is required. Transactions between female physicians and male nurses may be equally difficult in a culture where authoritative language typically has been transmitted from male to female.

Work-Family Conflict. Due to the time commitment required of physicians, substantial social/family pressure can be placed on balancing family commitments with professional responsibilities.

Personal Health. Physicians often are not willing to step outside their professional role to receive healthcare themselves. Physical and mental illness is no less prevalent among physicians than in the rest of the population. But the vulnerabilities of receiving care from colleagues, traditional risks to licensure with disclosures of certain medical conditions, and discomfort with the patient role create a tendency for physicians to avoid medical care.

OTHER IMPEDIMENTS TO PROGRESS

Porter and Teisberg[16] identified several technological, financial, and regulatory barriers that affect our healthcare system in the drive to improve *value-based competition.* Their notion of value is synonymous with CMS's initiatives to "transform itself from a passive payer of services into an active purchaser of higher quality, affordable care."[17] Porter and Teisberg's work permits an analysis of the intrinsic structural barriers to and opportunities for improved system design.

Technical

Society has changed with the influx of new technologies over the past half-century:

- While the first electronic medical record system was developed in the 1960s, extremely low rates of adoption of electronic medical records did not change until the Health Information Technology for Economic and Clinical Health Act (HITECH), enacted as part of the American Recovery and Reinvest Act of 2009, was passed to promote the adoption and meaningful use of health information technology.
- Social media that have emerged as a major communication medium came into existence in the past 20 years. Facebook was launched in 2004, Twitter in 2006, and TikTok in 2016.

- The International Statistical Classification of Diseases 10th Revision (ICD-10) became mandatory in the United States in 2013.
- Beepers and pager systems are becoming obsolete as healthcare providers adopt communication tools such as smartphones, personal digital assistants (PDAs), and iPads.
- Federal policy changes allowed widespread adoption of virtual televisits in 2020 as part of the response to the pandemic such that 76% of patients used telehealth services in 2020, an increase of 154% from the prior year.[18]

All of these technologies bring the promise of advancing care delivery, but they also challenge healthcare providers to keep pace with technological changes that may offer more efficient delivery of care than the current delivery system can accommodate.

The industry is transitioning from a state of intuitive medicine to a world of precision medicine enabled by the use of new diagnostic technologies and communication media. The impact of social media on healthcare delivery is yet to be fully realized or understood, but no doubt as younger physicians who grew up in a culture steeped in these media enter the profession, innovative ways of adopting these communication technologies for new patient care models will accelerate.

Ongoing Electronic Medical Record Challenges. In 2004 President George Bush issued a mandate for the nation's health system to work toward having electronic medical records in place in every hospital and doctor's office across the United States by 2014. The nation progressed but adoption was slow over the next four years.[19]

To accelerate the pace of adoption, in 2009, ARRA contained the HITECH Act, which set the foundation for the launch of CMS's Meaningful Use of Electronic Health Records program. This legislation provided the industry with more than $19 billion in incentive funding to put electronic medical records in place by 2015 for all eligible providers and facilities.

Currently, 89% of physicians have adopted EHRs; however, most EHR systems started out as billing systems and have been built on obsolete platforms designed to document based on fee-for-service governmental payment guidelines rather than user functionality.

By and large, physicians dislike EHRs and cite the lack of usability as a factor in physician burnout. *#LetDoctorsBeDoctors* is a movement sponsored by Athena Health that encourages healthcare professionals to express their frustration with laggard software and advocate for better technology.[20]

Ensuring that participating physicians and clinicians understand the potential *e-iatrogenic effect*[21] of these system changes (e.g., the potential for health information technology itself to cause harm) will be a crucial role for physician leaders to support goals for patient safety and quality of care.

On January 5, 2021, an amendment to the HITECH Act was signed into law requiring the U.S. Department of Health and Human Services "to consider certain recognized security practices of covered entities and business associates when making certain determinations, and for other purposes." This new law offers significant incentives for demonstrating to some unspecified degree the existence of recognized security practices.[22] Ongoing security issues with electronic health records have led to HIPAA regulatory requirements and penalties that further worsened the ease of access to essential information for patient care. The intention of the HITECH amendment is to ameliorate some of this impact.

Communication. The methods of communication involved in care delivery will change across traditional care settings and boundaries in the drive toward patient-centered care. In December 2006, the U.S. Supreme Court laid down new criteria on eDiscovery issued in the Federal Rules of Civil Procedure. These new rules affect health systems and physician practices by establishing the admissibility of electronic evidence in the court of law. *Twitter, Facebook,* and other social media tools were not mainstream at that time, but the evolution of communication tools is leading to several new electronic media sources being investigated in medico-legal cases.

Ownership of patient health data has been a concern for years due to the Health Insurance Portability and Accountability Act of 1996 (HIPAA). HIPAA and CMS' Meaningful Use rules from the HITECH Act of 2009 are driving the industry to increase abilities to exchange information more efficiently and securely while also making electronic patient records available to patients in their native format.

One of the technical barriers here lies in achieving a level of national interoperability across care settings and venues by achieving vendor platform interoperability. Patients need timely access to health information electronically, but the format in which this access is provided is still in development. Knowledge, reading level, native language, and technological capabilities among patients vary greatly, making standardization difficult. During the pandemic, access to telehealth varied by socioeconomic status, with new political debates centering on access to broadband capabilities as a social determinant of health that should be regulated like a public utility.[23]

Even within the context of the velocity of communication technology change, physicians are still ultimately on the front line with the patients and are held responsible as covered entities for stewardship over these data. Physician leadership, with its origination in the traditional physician duties of personal responsibility to the patient, must be an effective part of the management of medical information in the world of rapid change in communication technology.

Clinical Diagnostic Technologies. Advances in diagnostic technologies are providing new tools for physicians to help in the prevention and early detection of cancers, diabetes, respiratory conditions, and vascular diseases. These tools may have a transformative effect on healthcare delivery at the individual patient level and targeted populations; however, along with these advancements come new challenges.

Physicians are working to keep pace on the learning curve with these advancements in diagnostic capabilities. The field of molecular diagnostics alone has brought new laboratory testing options for physicians to order through the use of proteomics (protein analysis) and genomics (DNA analysis) laboratory technologies. Physicians in practice are challenged to stay current on an ever-increasing slate of technologies.

Meeting the requirements for clinical training to recognize what diagnoses warrant use of new tests, understanding reimbursement policies from payers, and interpreting test results all require accessing new knowledge on behalf of the individual physicians who are providing patient care services as well as those physician leaders in organizations working to make these new services available in their communities.

Comparative effectiveness information must interface with financial capital planning in a healthcare economy that is built on value. Effective point-of-care decision support tools with high usability must keep pace with diagnostic technologies, including advances in genomics, artificial intelligence, block chain, and other technologies on the horizon that will continue to impact patient care.

Education. Medical education is costly and is still most often provided in large academic medical centers, many of which are not adapting to the education techniques necessary for a future medical workforce.

In 2013, the American Medical Association created the Accelerating Change in Medical Education initiative, intended to jumpstart curricular and process changes and disseminate ideas on redesigning medical education. Citing the fact that health outcomes in underserved communities improve when physicians are more representative of the population who live there, the initiative is focused on policies to enhance and support medical student diversity. Initiatives also focus on developing a health system science to identify best practices in medical education, changing policy to support system-wide change, and facilitating team-based training and coaching. Future physicians are encouraged to develop adaptive skills and utilize them throughout their careers. [24]

Financial and Regulatory

The tremendous ongoing changes in the financial and regulatory arenas continue to present barriers that effective physician leaders need to address (Figure 2).

Fee-for-Service to Pay-for-Performance. A shift away from a volume-driven payment for services model to a future compensation system based on value and quality continues to develop. The 2015 passage of MACRA with overwhelming bipartisan support locked in the trajectory of the U.S. healthcare delivery system's move from one focused purely on fee-for-service revenue to one that increasingly required the demonstration of standards of quality.

The fee-for-service reimbursement system based on "transaction- and volume-based" healthcare makes no payment distinction between high or poor quality of care. Providers lose money if they reduce unnecessary service, whereas the actual services that can be provided are limited by specific fee codes and amounts.

These characteristics of fee-for-service led to several initiatives that move toward pay-for-performance models that include bundled payments, value-based purchasing, and incentive programs such as those we have emerging under the new accountable care organizations. However, for physician executives, a key barrier to leading their organizations through these financial reforms will be the transition to bearing greater risk for the quality of care delivered.

In the movement away from fee-for-service toward capitation and incentive-based reimbursement models, physicians assume a greater proportion of the risk for getting the right care delivered at the right time and at the right place. To be successful in the new payment systems, physicians and their organizations must turn toward delivering value and improving quality.

Potential Economic Impact
These technical, financial reform, and antitrust law issues are and will have multi-year effects on many health care organizations.

- **Technical.** While *near-term* costs for addressing these challenges have significant impacts to the health care system, the *long-term* benefits of improving quality of care should be the end goal of the investment.

- **Financial Reforms.** *Near-term* impact on physician practices and hospitals may be negative on revenue due to cultural transformation and change-over in reimbursement policies impacting revenue cycles.

- **Financial Reforms.** *Long-term* impact should result in stabilization of revenue streams for provider organizations and lower cost incurred by payers.

- **Antitrust.** *Near-term* impact on clinical integration joint ventures is for anticipated increased flexibility in safe harbors resulting in easing of requirements for accountable care organization formation.

- **Antitrust.** *Long-term* impact on market competition will have to be evaluated over time if integrated delivery networks continue to grow through acquisition of physician practices, ancillary care service providers, and facilities.

Figure 2.

Evidence-based medicine practices will play a greater role in clinical decisions with the use of clinical decision support tools to enhance the value of care delivered.

During the transition period, providers will be operating under two systems: some patients paid under fee-for-service and others under the pay-for-performance arrangement. Strong physician leadership will be important, as this change is at the heart of clinical decision-making and of accepting more of the burden of risk.

Antitrust Laws. Since the 1970s and 1980s, when mergers and consolidations in the industry started to accelerate, the Federal Trade Commission stepped-up enforcement activities, especially those construed to decrease competition involving physician practices (large or small), hospital organizations, and insurers. The Stark Law, Federal Anti-kickback Statute, and Certificate of Need activities have all been high management priorities in healthcare organizations for years, but the establishment of clinical integration processes is currently receiving the central focus and attention of physician leaders.

In 1996, the Federal Trade Commission issued its Statements of Antitrust Enforcement Policy in Health Care, which provided the legal framework by which various joint ventures between physician practices and hospital organizations have been and are evaluated. Clinical integration efforts are necessary to provide a solid foundation for the infrastructure development that will set the structure for process improvement.

Several criteria must be met for legal formation and operation that do not restrict trade or serve as a mechanism for financial kickback for referrals. The criteria include joint responsibility for substantial financial risk for quality outcomes among all involved parties. Safe harbors, especially in the case of accountable care organizations, will require some degree of alteration in current Federal Trade Commission policy to allow the diverse types of arrangements to form.

Systemic

Intrinsic challenges that transcend traditional boundaries and present as barriers to success for those physicians serving in leadership positions have developed over multiple generations, and the process of solving them or determining paths to work through them can be daunting.

System fragmentation and health policy reform are two facets of the same intrinsic challenges physician leaders must address.

System Fragmentation. The U.S. healthcare system is a highly fragmented delivery system. Exemplified by problems in coordination of care and access to care, the disparate nature of the system has created barriers for patients to receive the care they need and for physicians and other healthcare executives to make their own organizations and health system resources in the communities more efficient and effective.

The complexity of the delivery system, along with the lack of transparency in the payment system and lack of interoperability of health information systems, have created an environment in which neither free-market consumer-driven efficiencies nor single-payer cost containment strategies are effective.

Health Policy Reform. Health policy reform has a systemic effect at national, state, and local levels. Policy reform initiatives can take multiple iterations and phases over multi-year periods to achieve their strategic intent. However, when reforms at any of these levels produce negative impacts or unintended adverse consequences, the negative impact on physicians and other stakeholders can affect the goals of improved quality and accessibility of patient care. Historically, policy decisions in the U.S. have not been strongly influenced by physicians and other health professionals. Recently, a dramatic increase in the number of physician leaders engaged in collaborative activities to set policy direction is beginning to have an impact.[25]

Legislation such as the Social Security Act of 1965 that established the Medicare and Medicaid programs and the Health Maintenance Organization Act of 1973 that brought about significant change in the health insurance industry were intended to bring about sweeping positive effects for the health system. But for decades since the passage of these landmark acts, costs have continued to escalate. Some patients have received excellent care, others could not gain access to the care they needed.

Recognition of these barriers in the system as it is currently constructed has led to the new emphasis on a *patient-centered focus* in efforts to continue to refine the health system. In the 2010 Affordable Care Act, significantly more attention was placed on enacting changes that will place increased emphasis system-wide on strengthening patient-centered initiatives.[26] The 2015 MACRA act emphasized pay-for-performance and alternative payment model changes. The 21st Century Cures Act attempted to address information blocking and adopted a new health information technology certification requirement to enhance patients' smartphone access to their health information at no cost through the use of application programming interfaces. (APIs).[27] For physician leaders today, and those who will enter leadership in the future, engaging in policy formation decisions will be crucial to continuing to reduce these barriers for generations to come.

Physician leaders must help overcome the barriers that we face to optimize our nation's care delivery system. People and organizations resist change, but physician leaders must confront all intrinsic and extrinsic barriers to lead change in ways that effectively improve patient care.

REFERENCES

1. Our Ailing Medical System: It's Time to Operate the Medical Industrial Complex." *Fortune Magazine.* January 1970. New York: Harper & Row Library Catalog: MMS ID 99909393406676;NML ID 0256373.

2. Landi H. For First Time, Employed Physicians Outnumber Self-employed Doctors, AMA Study Finds. firecehealthcare.com, May 7, 2019.

3. Terry K. Why Health Systems Employ Doctors: Money and Control. *The Healthcare Blog*, August 31, 2020.

4. Curry W. *New Leadership in Health Care Management: The Physician Executive-Second Edition.* Tampa, FL: American College of Healthcare Executives, 1994. Chapter 6: The Dual Role Dilemma by Michael Kurtz, MS. pp. 81-88, Chapter

5: The Unique Contribution of the Physician Executive to Health Care Management by David Ottensmeyer, MD, FACPE and M.K. Key, PhD. p. 76.

5. Institute of Medicine (US) Committee on Quality of Health Care in America. *Crossing the Quality Chasm: A New Health System for the 21st Century*. Washington, DC: National Academies Press; 2001, pp. 25-33.

6. Rouse W. Health Care as a Complex Adaptive System: Implications for Design and Management. *The Bridge*. Spring 2008. pp. 17-25.

7. Bodenheimer T, Berry-Millett R. Follow the Money--Controlling Expenditures by Improving Care for Patients Needing Costly Services. *N Engl J Med*. 2009 Oct 15;361(16):1521-3.

8. Healthy People 2030. Health.gov.

9. Basen R. "It's Official: Med School Applications Well Up This Cycle," *Medpage Today*, January 7, 20201.

10. Howe K. *Where Have We Failed? A Systemic Analysis of U.S. Health Care*. Tampa Florida: American College of Physician Executives. 2002. p. 81.

11. Curry, p. 75.

12. Curry, p. 73.

13. Education Data. Average Medical School Debt. Educationdata.org. Accessed March 20, 2021.

14. Berg S. 5 Factors Contributing to Physician Stress During the Pandemic. *AMA Physician Health*. October 29, 2020.

15. Kane L. Medscape US and International Physicians'COVID-19 Experience Report: Risk, Burnout, Loneliness. Medscape. September 11, 2020.

16. Porter M, Teisberg E. *Redefining Health Care. Creating Value-Based Competition on Results*. Boston: Harvard Business Press; 2006, pp. 6-9, 218-219.

17. Centers for Medicare & Medicaid Services. Roadmap for Implementing Value Driven Healthcare in the Traditional Medicare Fee-for-Service Program. CMS Report. January 2009.

18. Wheel Team. Master Guide to Telehealth Statistics in 2020. Wheel.com. December 14, 2020.

19. Ford EW, Menachemi N, Peterson LT, Huerta TR. Resistance Is Futile: But It Is Slowing the Pace of EHR Adoption, Nonetheless. *J Am Med Inform Assoc*. 2009;16(3):274-281.

20. Versel N. What Do Physicians Hate About EHRs? *MedCity News*. February 2016.

21. Weiner JP, Kfuri T, Chan K, Fowles JB. E-Iatrogenesis: The Most Critical Unintended Consequence of CPOE and Other HIT. *J Am Med Inform Assoc*. 2007:14(3):387-8.

22. Mooney JA, Weinrich DA, Perkins LD. HITECH Act Amendment Offers New Incentive to Reduce Fines and Other Remedies. White and Williams LLP. January 11, 2021. www.whiteandwilliams.com/resources-alerts-HITECH-Act-Amendment-Offers-New-Incentive-to-Reduce-Fines-and-Other-Remedies.html.

23. Benda N, Veinot T Sieck C, Ancker J. Broadband Internet Access Is a Social Determinant of Health! *Am J Public Health*. 2020; 110(8):1123-5.

24. Smith T. Medical Education in 2020: How We Got Here, Where We're Headed Accelerating Change In Medical Education. AMA. March 17, 2020. www.ama-assn.org/education/accelerating-change-medical-education/medical-education-2020-how-we-got-here-where-we-re

25. Mclaughlin C, McLaughlin C. *Health Policy Analysis. An Interdisciplinary Approach.* Sudbury, MA: Jones and Bartlett Publishers; 2009, pp. 9-11.

26. United States Government. H.R. 3590, Patient Protection and Affordable Care Act, §6301(b). Establishment of Patient- Centered Outcomes Research Institute (2010); H.R. 3590, Patient Protection and Affordable Care Act, §3502(b)(4), Eligible entities for community health teams to support patient-centered medical homes (2010).

27. United States Government. HHS Extends Compliance Dates for Information Blocking and Health IT Certification Requirements in 21st Century Cures Act Final Rule, hhs.gov. October 29, 2020.

CHAPTER 4: BARRIERS TO HEALTHY CHANGE

Leadership Implications and Health Policy Considerations.

Leadership Implications:

1. Recognize the barriers to change that impact physician performance and professional satisfaction.
2. Engage in critical analysis of technology both as a disruptive innovation in a complex adaptive system and as return-on-investment from a patient-centered professional dialectic.

Health Policy Considerations:

1. When engaging in policy formulation, demonstrate broad understanding of the full magnitude of topics debated from economic, political, and social contexts while providing insight into their impact on the health of the community's population.
2. Support the need for additional research in how barriers to change impact physician well-being and limit effective leadership.

CHAPTER 5

We Started as Heroes

*Their lot has always been much the same. Hard work, long hours, poor accom-
modations for the majority, a sharp meeting with reality at a relatively young
age, a long grind of years — these have prevailed in every generation.*[1]

Earl P. Scarlett

From the earliest human literature derived from even earlier oral tradi-
tions of myth and legend, the figure of the hero is a recurring archetype. A young (usually male) adolescent is transformed by undergoing
a series of tests during a long journey. The hero endures physical challenges
others cannot withstand in order to save those unable to survive some ter-
rible ordeal on their own.

Heroes protect the weak and withstand enormous personal sacrifice for the
sake of an altruistic goal. Heroes are strong. They endure hardship. They succeed where others fail. Heroes save people.

In modern culture, superhuman action figures such as Superman and Bat-
man have superseded the mythological heroes of previous cultures. Hercules, St. Andrew, Florence Nightingale, Sergeant York are replaced with comic
book characters that are perceived as tongue-in-cheek parodies of previous
heroes from myth, legend, and history. Superman is nearly invincible: only
the occasional kryptonite brings him down to mere mortal power. He flies
and sees through buildings. Bullets bounce off him. He is never hungry,
sleepy, or sick. He overpowers enemies to save helpless victims.

In modern comic books, the superheroes are ageless, physically fit, and
hide their power with secret identities. They wear special uniforms and
hide behind masks and glasses until the need arises for their superhuman
transformation.

The similarities between these mythic cultural heroes and cultural expectations of the idealized physician are clear. Stereotypically, the physician's role
is to "save lives" without displaying personal suffering. The language and

culture of medical professionalism are used to mask the physician's emotions. The physician's white coat and scrubs are not a cape, tights, and boots, but they serve the same purpose of delineating a special identity for physicians that separates them from patients.

For a group of individuals in our society who endure its longest adolescent social role (student) in order to complete their professional training, physicians' identification with the role of hero could not be more enticing. The appeal of heroic mythology to adolescents coincides with the tension implicit in their transition from childhood to adult social roles. The lengthy apprenticeship of physicians extends adolescent transitional roles well into adulthood, such that physicians are culturally conditioned to identify with the role of hero and are trained to accept the value set of those presuming to take on this role.

A lifetime of delayed gratification, missed meals, sleep deprivation, and placing one's personal and family lives secondary to saving one's patients' lives becomes the social identity of the heroic physician. Doctors *fight* disease. They *save* lives. In the heroic language to describe physicians' professional lives, the implicit cultural expectation is that physicians perform this role with action, dispassion, and personal sacrifice.

Until recently, the dispassionate, self-sacrificing doctor who nonetheless acted in the patient's interest above their own was perceived as heroic due at least in part to personal sacrifice inherent in the acquisition of prolonged years of medical education and work hours required to be fully trained and professionally credentialed. Heroes do not whine or complain, and neither were doctors expected to do so.

Unfortunately, although they may seek to be perceived as invincible, physicians are susceptible to the same emotions and illnesses as other people. In a 2017 survey of 5,197 physicians, 44% reported symptoms of burnout using the Maslach Burnout Inventory, with a higher risk of burnout relative to other workers.[2] But those personifying the hero may hesitate to seek help.

Perhaps because they fear the loss of job security, 40% of physicians are reluctant to seek mental health treatment.[3] A study of female physicians found that only 6% of those with a mental health diagnosis reported it to their state licensing board; they stated they feared stigma.[4] Acknowledging lack of invincibility is inimical to the heroic persona that may be the etiology of the stigma they fear.

Physicians in contemporary American society are not unique in taking on the role of hero. The media images from the pandemic have focused on all frontline healthcare workers, nurses, and physicians equally. In 2020, nursing schools saw a 6% increase in applications, and medical schools saw an 18% increase.[5]

Twenty years ago, the uniformed firefighters who rushed into the World Trade Center were portrayed in the media as classic American heroes. Their personal sacrifice in their attempt to save the victims of the terrorist attack served as a catharsis for the nation by providing an inspiring counternarrative to the devastation wrought by the terrorists. Within days of the events of 9/11, black FDNY (Fire Department of New York City) t-shirts were worn all over the country, expressing a need to honor and identify with the heroes of the tragedy.

Typically, police officers and members of the military have been portrayed heroically, although events such as the torture and prisoner abuse by United States Army and Central Intelligence Agency personnel at Abu Ghraib early in the Iraq war and the murder of George Floyd by police officer Derek Chauvin in 2020 and have challenged these stereotypes.

In contrast to the national outrage generated by these horrific actions by individuals traditionally identified as heroes, the heroic physician image has not been similarly tarnished by media stories of individual physicians behaving atrociously. This image may be changing, however. The podcast and subsequent television series *Dr. Death* chronicling the gross negligence and sociopathic behavior of a Texas neurosurgeon has been popular. In addition, much of the pandemic anti-vax skepticism has been directed toward challenging physician goodwill and expertise.

Initiates can attain full recognition and initiation into the ranks of traditionally "heroic" professions such as nursing, firefighting, policing, or the military by their early 20s. In contrast, physicians, to quote a gastroenterologist colleague, "*give up an extra decade of their lives.*" Consequently, when they endeavor to take on the mantle of a board-certified, fully trained, and newly licensed physician, the medical initiate may be expecting a significant return on their investment of this "extra" decade of life.

As the high status of physicians has declined and financial compensation at the end of the training period has become less secure, some physicians have felt resentment and anger and acted out in disruptive ways. Others have focused their disappointment inwardly, where it may be manifested as depression, burnout, isolation, or hyper-criticality.

The impact of 7–12 years of training after four years of college begets an excessively prolonged social adolescence that especially acculturates physicians to identify with the hero role, including all of its limitations on behavior. Heroes have trained for action, not contemplation. The current fee-for-service payment model upon which most of the U.S. healthcare delivery system is built exacerbates these proclivities.

In the fee-for-service payment system, physicians are trained and paid for doing things. Surgeons make more money when they operate than when they don't. Doctors are paid well for cutting, scoping, diagnosing, prescribing, and testing, but not necessarily for listening or "watchful waiting." Health maintenance and preventive care codes have traditionally been difficult to get reimbursed.

Because the modern healthcare system trains its physicians for the role of hero, the cultural focus on action, superhuman sacrifice, and objectification of the patient as "victim" consequentially leads to an increase in healthcare costs. Failure to diagnose is now the most common malpractice claim. Watchful waiting confutes modern medicine's entire cultural and financial value system, which is based on action and heroic behavior.

In our culture, a hero's stereotypically expected reaction to barriers to action is anger and violence. Hercules breaks from his binding chains and lashes out at the enemy. By using force, he saves and helps. As the pressures our society faces from the rising economic costs of healthcare lead to measures to constrain physician behavior, one physician response is anger and lashing out.

The sacrificed "extra decade of life" in medical training no longer guarantees high status, high financial compensation, or freedom from restraints placed on others in society. The decision to operate or order a computed tomography (C.T.) scan may require prior authorization from a high school graduate sitting behind a computer at an insurance company. Regulation of physician behavior through the third-party payment system, increased oversight from non-physician membership on state medical boards, and hospital-based management of physician behavior through audit and peer review, like Hercules' chain, become barriers to the heroic propensity for unconstrained action.

In despair from the perceived futility of the sacrifice of the prolonged training period, physicians acting from the "heroic" archetype may choose to "break the chain" of constraints imposed on their autonomous actions. Unfortunately, if such action is directed at those in a physician's immediate environment in which the physician is working, rather than in attacking the inadequacies of the healthcare industry in systematic ways, the action will be labeled as "disruptive physician behavior."

In the operant conditioning of physician training, an easy role to assume under pressure is that of the "disruptive physician," as it is now called in healthcare administration literature. Disruption results from frustration with the healthcare system by someone trained to act, treat, and "attack" disease.

Entities attempting to control rising healthcare costs do not necessarily reward physicians for acting in the supposedly "super-heroic" role, nor do empowered healthcare consumers necessarily perceive themselves as victims in need of rescue by a doctor-hero. The common conflicts that pit hospital administration and insurance companies against physicians in the healthcare system lead to exploitation of the vulnerabilities of the "heroic" role physicians have been trained to assume.

Perhaps the inherent distaste physicians have expressed regarding pay-for-performance reimbursement reforms embraced by Medicare, managed care, and consumerist movements is partially a subconscious rejection of a non-heroic, objective measurement of worth as defined by the market.

Since the heroic role physicians assume will fail to be relevant in the future, physician training that focuses exclusively on heroic roles and actions will also fail to be relevant. Inevitably, physicians will respond to lower status and less compensation for heroic roles by changing their behavior patterns.

The partition of traditional comprehensive primary care roles into hospital-ists, SNFists, ambulatory specialists, telehealth specialists, and nocturnists allows primary care physicians to improve their lifestyles by practicing in a more limited setting. As physicians move to shift work, trade private practice for the security of employment contracts, wear scrub clothing indistinguish-able from other healthcare workers, their personification as heroes become less conspicuous.

Over time, physicians may no longer have a financial compensation advan-tage over other healthcare providers capable of delivering equally effective results. Current data indicate that advanced practice providers (APPs) achieve equivalent or better results on quality metrics and utilization com-pared to physicians. A 2018 Cochrane study of 18 randomized controlled tri-als suggested that nurse practitioners provide care equivalent to physicians and achieve similar patient outcomes in primary care settings.[6]

Most insurers reimburse for services provided by APPs at 85% of the rate paid to physicians. Physicians' incomes are generally higher due to this difference and the 30% higher number of patients seen relative to APPs. However, the compensation differential does not make up for the difference in training requirements for a physician compared to a nurse practitioner or physician assistant. Nurses must complete at least 1,000 hours of clinical practice in a focused area, such as pediatric, adult, or geriatric medicine, to earn an NP degree. Physician assistants train for two years and complete at least 2,000 hours of supervised practice before graduation.

In contrast to NPs and PAs, a typical family physician completes 15,000 hours of clinical work over five additional years of training, including residency,[7] although questions remain regarding the quality, efficiency, and cost-effectiveness of care provided by physicians and APPs in different care settings and among complex patient populations.[8] However, the personal cost of obtaining a full medical license as a physician rather than APP is substantially higher both financially and in years of training and on average results in substantially more personal debt.

Ultimately, physicians expect a social and financial return on investment for their extensive training relative to other healthcare professionals. But the traditional role of hero implies self-sacrifice. Lack of insight by society into the nuanced interplay of expected return on investment both financially and in terms of status needs to be acknowledged. The public's lack of empathy for physicians' financial indebtedness and poor compensation during training is part of the inherent conflict with changing social expectations.

The interplay of the social dynamics of the economic laws of supply and demand with the cultural expectation of altruism in heroic figures will force physicians to choose a different role. If physicians' tasks can be done by other healthcare providers who require less training, improved with point-of-care decision support and evidence-based protocol, the unique status of physicians will need to be built on something other than the traditional heroic archetype.

Physicians will need to metamorphose from a heroic role to one based on leadership to maintain high status. Physicians will need to acquire the training of the management disciplines and responsibilities of governance to conserve their professional preeminence in healthcare. The integrated healthcare delivery model will require leadership training in medicine, management, information systems, and systems analysis. Such physicians will continue to shape the patient's medical experience through a knowledge base and experience acquired over a prolonged training period.

The demand for a healthcare system that meets patients' needs with compassion, efficiency, and high quality may be a tall order for those trained within a context based on a cultural identity focused on the heroic archetype. It will acquire additional acculturation into a more socially mature leadership role.

THE HEROIC MODEL OF CONTEMPORARY TRAINING

Medical students are selected for and trained in certain characteristics and behaviors that develop their professional identity within the context of the heroic model. When it is successful, medical education should amalgamate these traits into a unified level of technical and emotional competence required to fulfill the professional role in which physicians are empowered in the current U.S. healthcare system.

Academic Excellence. First, the extensive education for physicians requires *academic excellence* specifically to develop analytical, critical thinking, and communication skills in addition to clinical knowledge. Individuals who become physicians are typically drawn from the top 5% of students in American colleges. The ability to perform well in the classroom, excellent performance on standardized tests, exceptional memorization skills, and top grades in mathematics and the sciences are core competencies that medical schools look for among those competing for admission.

Perseverance. The second characteristic is *perseverance*. Physician training requires years of study, an extensive clinical knowledge base, and a pathophysiological approach to diagnosing and treating disease that is learned over a prolonged period of didactic training and experiential learning. Individuals who eventually earn the degrees of Doctor of Medicine or Doctor of Osteopathy have typically spent four years in college, four years in medical school, and 3–12 years in postgraduate training before achieving full licensure in their specialties.

Delaying Gratification. Third is the *capacity to delay gratification*. The professional rewards of high status, authority, respect, and potential for high financial compensation as a practicing physician are delayed until full licensure. Any freshly minted MD/DO in an internship can tell a personal story of caring for patients all night long, only to have an anxious family member demand to talk to the *real* doctor as soon as possible.

Medical education requires the ability to delay gratification for years of effort in the education and training process before receiving status and full professional authority. In their day-to-day lives, medical students and physicians are expected to delay gratification of their personal needs in their attempts to meet the needs of patients. At the physical level, it is as mundane as suppressing the need to empty one's bladder, sleep, or eat during a medical emergency or rushed patient schedule.

Self-abnegation. A fourth trait expected of physicians is *self-abnegation* in order to fulfill the expected ethical and moral obligations based on the altruism of the physician in the doctor-patient relationship. More than simply delaying gratification, such self-denial is forgoing any personal reward if it interferes with what is in the patient's best interests.

The American Medical Association's Code of Medical Ethics lays this out as a specific responsibility: "A physician shall, while caring for a patient, regard responsibility to the patient as paramount."[9]

Specifically, "The relationship between a patient and a physician is based on trust, which gives rise to physicians' ethical responsibility to place patients' *welfare above the physician's own self-interest or obligation to others*, to use sound medical judgment on patients' behalf, and to advocate for their patients' welfare."[10]

The pre-medical student who skips the fraternity party to study for an organic chemistry exam, the medical student who turns down a date in order to prepare for board exams, and the intern who stays by the bedside of a dying patient rather than going home to her toddler's birthday party are not simply delaying gratification; they are choosing to forgo certain experiences obligated in their professional role.

Implicit in the expectation that physicians will forgo such personal pleasures for the sake of their education and patient care is the altruistic value upon which the physician-patient relationship is based and in the high status granted to physicians for making these sacrifices.

Suppressing Revulsion. A fifth trait necessary for physicians is being *capable of suppressing revulsion.* The human aspects of patient care required of healthcare professionals are apparent from the cadavers present on the first day of medical school. Physicians cannot omit the carnal experience of medicine from their daily professional experience.

Everyone in direct healthcare is involved with the physical aspects of human disease, whether it is the nursing assistant emptying a bedpan or the surgeon amputating a gangrenous limb. But it is not a part of the professional experience of most other highly educated and high-status professionals, such as attorneys, healthcare administrators, investment bankers, or academic professors. Physicians have a unique place among the highest status professionals in being exposed to these corporeal aspects of the human experience.

Squeamish college students contemplating medical school had best set their sights on alternative careers.

These five traits may be seen as essential to contemporary medical training in order to develop medical students within the heroic model of the physician profession. They are essential but not comprehensive; within the broader context of leadership training of physicians, these traits do not address the inherent problems of physicians as autonomous decision-makers (heroes) versus leaders of teams within organized systems of care.

Thus, medical training requires a reorganization around other essential traits to develop appropriate leadership capacity in physicians, including effective communication skills, change management skills, strategic (rather than just tactical) thinking, and effective teamwork. Empathy is as important as self-abnegation, and excellent communication is as crucial as academic excellence. Resilience must balance perseverance in a team environment.

THE HEROIC ACADEMIC JOURNEY

Becoming a doctor requires a series of complex personal choices be made in a relatively brief period of time regarding one's self-identity in the confusing environment of medical school. Having survived the coursework and testing required for medical school admission, the medical student is typically rushed into a fact-oriented curriculum of anatomy, biochemistry, microbiology, pharmacology, physiology, and histology. Subsequently, after some course work in physical diagnosis, medical students rotate through a series of clinical clerkships designed to expose them to various forms of medical practice. In two-month blocks, pediatrics, internal medicine, general surgery, obstetrics and gynecology, family medicine, and psychiatry are completed in rapid succession.

Rapid shifts in demographics, science, and federal policies, are changing the education and training of physicians. Multiple initiatives are underway to better identify and implement processes and policies that improve medical education. Over the past 10 years, medical schools have begun testing how to select students with personal characteristics that allow them to work in teams, interact with diverse people, be resilient, adapt to different situations, and think critically.[11]

Additionally, the AAMC-sponsored MCAT has added two new sections to the existing biological science content covering critical thinking as well as behavioral and social sciences. Many schools are enhancing instruction on population health, addiction, communication skills, social determinants of health, and medical informatics. Recent reform efforts are focused on fully integrated curricula where basic and clinical sciences are integrated with health systems science and a broader biopsychosocial model of health.[12]

Some schools are integrating coursework in medical professionalism and leadership early on, but these formal curriculum changes must consider the environment in which the students are trained. Within the prolonged period of physician training is a significant "foxhole" effect. Medical students, interns, residents, and fellows are all immersed in their wearying experience together, often spending more time with one another than they do with their own family members.

Similar to the attitude of enlisted soldiers about their officers, medical students and residents may identify with one another more than with faculty physicians. Their peers influence their behavior more than do their teachers at points in the experiential learning process. *"See one; do one; teach one"* is the educational model of medical procedure education and is based on the interaction between the students and house staff, not necessarily with the teaching faculty. The shaping of professionalism occurs in the trenches among peers.

During medical school, students are expected to choose a specialty because they typically spend the final year of medical school focused on more specialized rotations within the broader fields. Future urologists, dermatologists, anesthesiologists, or radiologists might get a crack at a clerkship in these fields as a fourth-year student while they are also bustling to show their work ethic in a sub-internship in their anticipated field of study and interviewing with residency programs for choice postgraduate spots.

In this environment, the students who are working to distinguish themselves from their fellow students exchange information informally while simultaneously relying on one another to understand proper behavior on the wards.

The importance of the informal curriculum in every medical school and teaching hospital environment in shaping professional behavior must be understood in order to positively impact leadership training.[13] The informal curriculum is about the culture, structure, and processes that form each academic medical institution. The communication dynamics within the informal curriculum, to a greater or lesser extent, shape the student's experience. Each individual medical school and graduate training program has its own culture that has evolved over time, so incorporating new elements of medical training will need to be developed within the context of the unique culture of each education program.

With the renewed industry focus on professionalism and recognition of a greater need for emphasis on managerial and communication skills for physician leaders, every medical school in the nation will need to understand the informal culture in which its medical education occurs and address potential derailers of the new curricular requirements.

Like every other American institution, U.S. medical school education has radically changed since the first medical school opened in 1765 at the University of Pennsylvania. Advances in therapeutics and diagnostics through pharmaceuticals, medical technologies, surgical techniques, biotechnologies, and rapidly advancing fields of genomics and proteomics have pushed clinical knowledge of the human body and the ability to impact disease far beyond what any of our nation's earliest physician leaders could have ever imagined.

American medical schools have produced some of the top physicians across the clinical, scientific, and leadership spectrum. However, contemporary academic medical institutions face substantial challenges in preparing future physicians for practice and leadership roles that will meet the needs of the rapidly evolving healthcare delivery system.

Medical school leaders face a complex and growing set of competing priorities in the need to meet research obligations, educate medical students through experiential learning, generate adequate revenue to fund training programs, and, most importantly, advance the medical culture focused on quality improvement and patient safety through clinical training of interns and resident physicians.[14]

However, these institutional needs originating from the processes, culture, and organizational framework of academic medical institutions do not mesh seamlessly with the overall political and social agendas of current healthcare reform efforts. Coupled with the ongoing transformation of primary care, specialty care, and hospital environments during the past several decades, needs for new, experiential learning models for medical students in clinical clerkships continue to challenge the infrastructure, financial business models, and culture of traditional academic medical institutions.

For example, the traditional medical school approach to education through core foundational knowledge in anatomy, physiology, pathology, biochemistry, and the other natural medical sciences, followed by clerkships in the traditional medical specialties requiring the diagnostic skill set emphasized in the 20th-century healthcare system (e.g., anesthesiology, radiology, vascular interventions) is hard-pressed to keep pace with the emergence of medical specialties based on place of service (e.g., emergency medicine, hospitalists, urgent care), or form of service (e.g., medical home, retail clinics, virtual medicine, ambulatory intensive care units).[15]

The convergence of these priorities creates new pressures for the traditional culture of medical training to prepare future physicians more appropriately for clinical practice and leadership roles in the healthcare system. The foundation of clinical knowledge and experiential learning that is needed to support their chosen specialty areas and development of the necessary skill sets of particular medical specialties must be rich enough and fluid enough to permit expertise in diagnosis and assessment of a patient while deriving plans of care based upon medical evidence within the context of accurate interpretation of various environmental, social, and behavioral factors that may contribute to the patient's status.

During the long years of training, they must also develop technical proficiency in specialty-specific medical procedures and diagnostic techniques. Additionally, attention is needed to strengthen the physician's leadership abilities. The skills of communication, team-building and motivation, resource allocation, and strategy and planning will be equally important to lead healthcare organizations through their current transformation.

The weaknesses of the current medical education system in addressing physician leadership development for healthcare organizations in a value-based economic model require appropriate delineation and analysis in order to close the gaps inherent in the current institutional structure and culture.

THE ECOSYSTEM FOR TRAINING HEROES

In 1910, at the behest of Dr. Henry Pritchett of the Carnegie Foundation and the American Medical Association, Abraham Flexner traveled throughout the United States and Canada to visit 150 medical schools and returned to publish *Medical Education in the United States and Canada*. He evaluated entrance requirements, size and training of faculty, the sum of endowment and fees, quality and adequacy of laboratories and teachers, and relations between the schools and hospitals.

Flexner's formal accusation of uncontrolled proprietary medical schools turning out masses of poorly trained physicians for profit led to the complete reorganization of medical education and the closing of hundreds of for-profit proprietary schools. He advocated minimal admission standards, standard curriculums of study, natural sciences, laboratory and clinical training, and warned of the danger of a crowded curriculum:

... [M]edical curricula the world over contain too many subjects as well
as too much material. ... Men become educated by steeping themselves
through a few subjects, not by nibbling at many.[16]

He stressed the importance of biological science, which is now the basis of
present-day medical curricula. However, much of Flexner's insights into the
dual role of the physician as arbiter in both the biological and social sciences
have been underemphasized in medical school curricula, which thus com-
pounds other inherent weaknesses in the training culture:

The physician's function is fast becoming social and preventive, rather than
individual and curative. Upon him society relies to ascertain ... and enforce
the conditions that prevent disease and make positively for physical and
moral wellbeing.[17]

The Flexner report's impact on medical education in the United States was
profound. It focused on standardizing medical education, but its inherent
racial and gender biases have had a lasting impact. After the report, all but
66 schools shut down, including five of seven Black medical schools and six
of seven women's medical colleges.

Flexner wrote that African-American physicians should be trained in "hygiene
rather than surgery" and should primarily serve as "sanitarians," whose purpose was "protecting whites" from common diseases like tuberculosis.[18] He
argued that there was no need for medical school specifically devoted to
women and recommended that all such schools be closed. He explained that
"it is clear that women show a decreasing inclination" to enter the profession
because "any strong demand for women physicians or any strong ungratified
desire on the part of women to enter the profession ... is lacking."[19]

In streamlining and standardizing medical education, Flexner's report transformed medical doctors into well-respected professionals with extensive
and complex training, but also constructed upon an ideal medical student
prototype of "northern wealthy white men whose "professional patriotism"
(heroism) is best cultivated with a more homogenous pool of doctors who
are deserving the subsequent societal privileges they should be" given.[20]

The adoption of Flexner's recommendations for a standardized curriculum
narrowed medical education in terms of race, sex, and social class. Simultaneous, the post-Flexner curricula had intrinsic systemic weaknesses due to
never integrating Flexner's original vision of educating physicians for their
social and preventive roles:

The reconstruction of medical education on the basis of two years of
required college work is not, however, going to end matters once and for

all. It leaves untouched certain outlying problems that will all the more surely come into focus when the professional training of physicians is more securely established on a scientific basis. At that moment, the social role of the physician will generally expand. And to support such expansion, the physician will crave a more liberal and disinterested educational experience. The question of age—not thus far important because hitherto our demands have been well within the limits of adolescence—will now require to be reckoned with. The college freshman averages 19 years of age. Two years of college will permit him to begin the study of medicine at age 21, to be a graduate at 25, to get a hospital year and begin practice at age 26 or 27.[21]

Thus, Flexner recognized the dual problem of the prolonged period of training necessary for adequate medical education and the need for a broader, more liberal education to fulfill the expanded social role of the physician, even if his racial and gender biases diminished his ability to see individuals who were not white males as adequate initiates into the profession.

In *Time to Heal*, Ludmerer identifies weaknesses in the non-clinical training of physicians that have diminished the quality of medical education experienced from the time of Flexner's report to the era of managed care. These inherent weaknesses include a culture of student abuse, faculty pressure for research and publishing, and the impact of insurance and managed care upon teaching.[22]

After the Flexner report, medical education became firmly established in the academic centers, and a significant emphasis on the physical sciences became normative. Funding of medical research through the academic medical schools accelerated with the establishment of the Medicare and Medicaid system in the 1960s and, with it, the attention of faculty to prioritize research over teaching and patient care.

Whereas the vast majority of clinical training occurs in the inpatient arena, the Health Maintenance Organization Act in 1973 placed pressure on medical institutions to limit hospitalized patients' length of stay and move procedures to the ambulatory setting. Superimposed managed care gatekeeper models reduced the status of generalists and pushed students into the more financially lucrative specialties requiring a larger number of years in training. Although these changes launched new ways of conducting the business of healthcare, little classroom preparation for the business aspect of medicine exists in standard curricula.

Medical student abuse. The competitive nature of medical school admissions, the need to train physicians in the ethics of putting the needs of patients before their own, and the captive and isolating nature of the prolonged period of medical training have fostered a culture of abuse during the clinical training and residency years. Verbal abuse is the type most frequently reported, but other forms of abuse also occur, given the position of power and authority of those supervising and overseeing the efforts of third- and fourth-year medical students. As a result of abuse, medical students face a number of distresses that include anxiety, unnecessary stress, burnout, and depression.[23]

While medical schools have acknowledged this problem and many have taken steps to eradicate it, the Association of American Medical Colleges' (AAMC) graduation questionnaire administered annually to all 140 allopathic medical schools indicates more than one-third of respondents reported experiencing at least one type of mistreatment, with the most common form of mistreatment being public humiliation, reported by 21.1% of survey respondents in 2017.

Analysis of these data indicated nearly twice as many lesbian, gay, or bisexual students reported an episode of mistreatment compared to heterosexual students (43.5% vs. 23.6%), and 40.9% of female students reported an episode of mistreatment compared to 25.2% of male students. Reports of mistreatment were higher for Asian (31.9%), underrepresented minority (38.0%), and multiracial (32.9%) students compared to white students (24.0%).[24]

Given the long-term ramifications that such abuse can have on the practicing physician, changing the medical school and teaching hospital cultures to eliminate these occurrences should be a top priority to secure the health and well-being of future physicians and medical community leaders.

Faculty pressure for research and publishing. The post-World War II academic medical center is financially differentiated from the rest of the healthcare delivery system by cross-subsidization from federal funding for teaching, but more extensively by federal and commercial research grants. Thus, the pressure on medical school faculty to produce an ever-increasing amount of research to advance their careers often trumps any emphasis on their teaching roles.

As financial pressures have mounted on academic medical centers to find additional funding sources, opportunities to secure funding through grant research programs from the National Institutes of Health (NIH) and other federal and state agencies have steadily increased over the past five decades. However, one of the most critical negative impacts is the decreased attention and time dedicated by top faculty to teach. This trend affects both classroom training and experiential learning by limiting the time afforded by clinical faculty members to provide feedback and counseling to medical students, clinical clerks, and residents. In such an environment, mentoring to shape critical, clinical, and communication skills is not optimized.

Insurance and managed care impact. The managed care strategy to drive down the per-unit cost of care results in an increase in the volume necessary for profitability, leaving less time for teaching and more scrutiny of the quality of care by payers, who do not see it as their responsibility to subsidize the higher costs of care associated with academic medical centers.

There is little room in the high-volume, low-unit-cost world of managed care reimbursement for the cost of teaching and training the next generation of healthcare providers. That function, although cross-subsidized by research and federal grants, does not enhance the bottom line, and is underinvested by private industry payers. Managed care increased pressure to maximize the productivity of physicians in the teaching hospital environment just as it does in other settings.

In the 1990s, at the same time the fee-for-service system increased the emphasis on volume and productivity, Medicare payments to fund residency positions were reduced. Cuts in funding and pressures on faculty to see a higher volume of patients and/or generate more revenue from clinical research certainly constrained medical education and exacerbated the underlying potential for exploitation and abuse inherent in the prolonged apprenticeship of medical education.

NEW PARADIGM FOR LEARNING

The socioeconomic changes of the 20th century co-evolved with a technological and information revolution that is beginning to transform medical care. Just as society's needs for medical care have changed, so have medical students' interests in selecting specialty areas for career choices to focus on during their medical education.

In recent decades, several specialty areas have grown in popularity[25] while primary care field disciplines such as internal medicine and family medicine have declined postgraduate training enrollment. Starr noted that from the mid-20th century, underlying structural factors in the healthcare industry contributed to the rise of physician specialization, including:[26]

- The system for certifying medical specialists was not regulated to a degree of capping or monitoring the number or distribution of specialists in any given field.

- After World War II, substantial incentives received by hospitals to set up clinical training programs for specialists increased the supply.
- A high financial return on investment for remaining in fellowship specialty training for two to three years longer through higher reimbursement from payers encouraged specialization in procedure-focused fields.

Consequently, the industry is significantly challenged to keep pace with the demand for primary care physician services to meet the needs of the aging baby boomer population for decades to come.[27]

The Council on Graduate Medical Education (COGME) has assessed over the past decade, issues of demand versus supply of primary care and specialty physicians and how academic medical schools have worked to address or meet market needs.[28] Early career direction-setting of physicians has been partially guided by where students saw market demand for their services coupled with their intrinsic desires and skills. The academic medical center's high-acuity, highly specialized research and tertiary care work environment does not provide an abundance of primary care role models for medical students, nor are primary care physicians venerated or awarded high status in such institutions.

As a growing need for developing a stronger foundation of managerial, communication, and business acumen will be required across the spectrum of specialty care, physicians will be required to operate from a more entrepreneurial context in traditional independent/group practices, virtual environments, and larger institutional settings. Foundational skills in management and communication can sharpen the entrepreneurial mindset that helps create pathways to validate and accelerate use of innovations, ensure the application of evidence-based medicine practices, and enhance physician leaders' abilities to develop new ways to reduce cost and improve the quality of care. Regardless of the specialty chosen, physicians trained in these foundational skills will be more likely to become successful leaders.

Porter and Teisberg identify some of the critical skills that will be important in medical education moving forward, including multidisciplinary teaming, knowledge management, an understanding of integrated care culture and processes, and stronger training in health informatics tools.[29]

Physician practices have been changing over the past two decades from the autonomous model of operation to newer and more clinically integrated models that require physicians to be skilled at collaborative decision-making and comfortable with distributed authority. With the emergence of clinically integrated networks, integrated delivery systems, and accountable care organizations, having strong managerial and communication skills is rapidly becoming a prerequisite for physicians to navigate and help steer organizations.

In 2004, the IOM's Committee on Behavioral and Social Sciences in Medical School Curricula recommended that all medical schools should develop and offer an *"integrated 4-year curriculum in the behavioral and social sciences"*[30] in which two of the key domains were the physician's role and behavior and health policy and economics. Focus on topics such as economic incentives, cross-functional teamwork, and social accountability were identified as critical domains in medical education.

The committee acknowledged the importance of effective communication skills not only for patient-physician relations but to help strengthen medical students' and physicians' abilities to relate to other physicians and multidisciplinary colleagues across the spectrum of the healthcare operating environment.

More recently, the American Medical Association has created its Accelerating Change in Medical Education initiative that is focused on disseminating innovation to better train physicians to meet the needs of patients today and in the future. The AMA is working with a consortium of academic training centers to develop an approach to medical education reform based upon newer approaches to learning and competencies:

- **Developing flexible, competence-based pathways**: Medical education is shifting away from classrooms and toward activities and assessments that help students succeed in the modern healthcare system.
- **Teaching new content in health systems science**: Medical schools are focusing on improving healthcare quality, delivering population-based medical care, and establishing healthcare teams by teaching health systems science.
- **Working with healthcare delivery systems in novel ways**: Medical schools are partnering with healthcare systems to bring students out of classrooms to learn in authentic healthcare settings.
- **Making technology work for learning**: Medical education is focusing on adapting technology in new ways to solve key problems and advance physician training, such as the use of electronic health records, management of patient panels to improve health outcomes, and interpretation of "big data" on healthcare costs and utilization.
- **Envisioning the master adaptive learning**: Medical schools are preparing today's medical students for careers in the changing healthcare system

that requires more than clinical skills by modeling how physicians must continually learn, adjust and innovated as new information and best practices evolve.

• **Shaping tomorrow's leaders**: The participating consortium schools are integrating leadership and teamwork training into curricula to prepare students to become future leaders.[31]

These reform efforts have in common a recognition that the standardized science-based curriculum that arose after the Flexner report is no longer adequate for today's students' professional needs. As Wiley Souba MD, former dean of Dartmouth's Geisel School of Medicine, puts it:

> The new themes that increasingly have to be part of medical education raise a host of interesting question. For example, what does it mean to be a leader—whether you are in solo practice, as large group practice, or a large academic health center? How do you measure how you are doing in your practice? How do you provide the best care of the highest quality at the lowest cost? . . . How do you rebound from bad news or a bad outcomes: There is a need to create infrastructure that allow for better alignment of medical education inside the professional nature of healthcare.[32]

The paradigm shift that integrates clinical, social, and behavioral sciences into the medical curriculum is the common thread present in all of these proposed curriculum redesign efforts a century after Flexner recommended such an approach. Medical students hone their diagnostic and critical thinking skills in all three of these basic sciences, growing in their ability to assess, interpret, act, and direct efforts of patient care teams and influence the actions of patients through physician ordering and recommendations.

The success of a patient-centered culture embedded in the medical home and accountable care models will depend on such paradigm shifts in medical education.

SPECTRUM OF MOTIVATIONS

All people operate consciously in one of three states of motivation at any moment in time. People are either focused on *survival*, on *pleasure*, or on the *existential meaning* of their lives. For an individual, these three states of motivation can be altered instantaneously by external events.

Consider, for example, how quickly a pleasant drive on a sunny day can alter someone's motivation by a sudden need to swerve to avoid a collision. For physicians in training, these three states of conscious motivation can be continually intermingled.

Most medical students have elevated levels of financial indebtedness. They may suppress ordinary personal physical, mental, or spiritual needs for the sake of patient care. Many physicians, extremely good at delaying gratification, get through their training years with irregular meals and irregular sleep patterns. The motivation to have a meaningful existence within the physician professional role may authenticate the altruism necessary to place the needs of patients above their own needs.

Physicians in training expect security and high status once they complete their training. During training, students begin treating patients but do not have any special status. Nonetheless, there is an expectation of modeling behavior built on self-sacrifice as a professional standard. As medical students, interns, residents, and fellows move through their training curriculum, a professional self-awareness of where one is operating at any moment in time regarding these three motivational states could become part of the contemporary medical culture.

Traditionally, medical trainees have been expected to push through nights on call, workdays with no sleep, poor meals, inadequate exercise, and verbal abuse from those in power. Awareness of the complexity of one's motivational state may offer the unreflective physician community a philosophical language in which to articulate the stresses inherent in the bifurcation of personal versus professional identity. Concomitant in the drama of "becoming a doctor" are expectations of serving as the healer who makes personal sacrifices.

Physician training does not particularly engender the development of empathy, but it can be linked more so to the *existential meaning* of the physician's chosen career path. Physicians are trained to maintain a level of professional detachment from their patients in order to be objective. There is a need for detachment simply to get through the training experience.

From the first month of medical school, they are exposed intimately to death through the dissection of cadavers. As most medical training occurs in tertiary medical centers where the sickest and most complex patients are, their first pediatric rotations will likely be on a hematology/oncology ward or a neonatal intensive care unit where young children are dying. The autopsies they participate in as second-year pathology students may be on young adults, such as themselves, as teaching institutions seek to learn about the premature death of the young by pushing for an autopsy evaluation much more vigorously than one would experience in a community setting.

The tension between professional detachment and empathy may lead to suppression of awareness of personal suffering. This suppression may allow

Four Paths of the Corporate Soul

Izzo and Klein's concept offered a framework for "leaders and companies to consider in creating soul and commitment in the workplace."

1. **Path of Self.** A heightened awareness of one's passion and values and the opportunity for leaders to create workplace environments that welcome this attribute.

2. **Path of Contribution.** People start to recognize the critical meaning of their work. Understanding the value of our contributions to achieving desired outcomes.

3. **Path of Craft.** Focus on the ongoing process of learning and mastery of a skill that brings about an awareness of previously unknown skills.

4. **Path of Community.** Where individuals come together with others and find opportunities to grow both individually and collectively for the benefit of society.

Figure 1.

a medical trainee to function in the role of healer and offer some degree of psychological self-protection. The need for the informal cultures of medical schools to incorporate values inherent in effective teamwork, systems theory, and business acumen that takes place within an environment in which empathy, inspirational leadership, and enhanced self-awareness are pivotal educational experiences can serve to transform the heroic model of medical education, with its focus upon denial of personal suffering in the physician role, to one in which there is a healthier balance between one's personal and professional identity.

Izzo and Klein developed the concept of the *"four paths to corporate soul"*[33] from their efforts to help organizations and their leaders understand how to tap into the "inner soul" of themselves as leaders and the members of their organizations (Figure 1).

Within the context of the need for change in the curriculum and informal culture of medical education, their four paths may offer a way of incorporating appropriate leadership training into professional development by creating the categories by which necessary competencies can be assessed.

Assessment of physicians in training in *self-awareness, contribution, craft,* and *community* may provide a framework to guide academic medical institutions to more effective models of professional training. A focus on the development of a healthy way of living and as assessed through the four paths defined by Izzo and Klein should improve physician performance both as leaders and competent clinicians.

AN INFLECTION POINT

The culture, environment, and processes of medical education are an example of a *complex adaptive system*. Efforts to strengthen the healthcare system will succeed only if we recognize the complexity of its characteristics and dynamic elements.

Self-organization is one trait of complex adaptive systems that must be understood in order to approach medical education reform in both the formal and informal curricula of academic medical institutions. The ability of the healthcare industry to restructure, reorganize, and set new priorities in order to meet community needs will require a sustainable model of medical education that can thrive as part of a broader complex adaptive system.

A transformation of the physician role from hero to a more resilient one that can be assessed within the context of *self-awareness* (of one's professional role, personal needs, and personal strengths and weaknesses), *contribution* (to the health and well-being of patients), *craft* (the art and clinical skills of the practice of medicine), and *community* (in one's role in providing leadership, being a member of a healthcare team, and improving the overall health of the population) will help support the establishment of this new model.

Physicians who are assessed within this context should have strengthened skills in what Bohmer identifies as "operations design, negotiation and conflict resolution, team management, and human resources and data management."[34] The need for these types of skills provides a basis for instituting education in organizational management and healthcare policy in the medical education of clinicians at all levels of training and practice. Moreover, failure to do so will deprive physicians of the ability to understand and communicate with the other "actors" in the healthcare arena.[35]

Healthcare legislation in the past few years recognized the need to provide an infusion of funding and new programs to support physician and health professional education. Section 5101 and 5301 of the Affordable Care Act established the National Healthcare Workforce Commission and Training in Family Medicine, General Internal Medicine, General Pediatrics, and Physician Assistantship. The National Healthcare Workforce Commission established a 15-member chartered commission from across the spectrum of stakeholders in our nation's health system whose focus will be:

- To evaluate healthcare education and training activities to ensure that demand for healthcare workers and physicians is being met.
- To identify barriers to improve coordination of healthcare education across federal, state, and local levels.
- To support ideas for innovation with the potential to address population health needs, changes in technology, and other environmental factors.

The primary care training enhancement program (Section 5301) authorizes DHHS to provide grant and contract funding to accredited public or non-profit private hospitals, schools of allopathic or osteopathic medicine, academically affiliated physician assistant training programs, or other public or private not-for-profit entities focused on physician education and training. The purpose of this program is to improve the formal and informal curricula for such institutions, add to the number of funded residencies and internships, provide new financial assistance to medical students for fellowships or traineeships, and provide additional funding to support physicians who elect to teach in the programs specified under this section of the legislation.

In the Consolidated Appropriations Act of 2021, Congress established 1,000 new Medicare-supported graduate medical education positions, the first such increase in 25 years. The AAMC is currently leading efforts to establish 14,000 new Medicare graduate medical education slots over seven years, particularly focused on hospitals in rural areas, in states with new medical schools, and in areas with health professional shortages.

The traditional strengths of our medical education system have been rooted in our clinical training for medical students, interns, and residents. Several universities have established dual degree programs for physicians to obtain master's degrees in business administration or management disciplines along with others to help enhance their business acumen and managerial and communication skills.

But more effort is needed. As Abraham Flexner suggested a century ago, social and behavioral science education for physicians will help drive the effectiveness of innovations in care delivery design that will improve outcomes in patient care across the country. The renewed focus on building capacity in our nation's physician and health professional workforce through improved support to the medical education system has the potential to mitigate some of the health system's current challenges; improve operational efficiency and effectiveness; and, in the long run, yield improved patient outcomes as long as it simultaneously adapts the physician role to one that is healthy and sustainable for both doctors and patients.

REFERENCES

1. Scarlett E. *In Sickness and In Health: Reflections on the Medical Profession.* Toronto: McClelland & Stewart; 1972.

2. Shanafelt TD, West Cp, Sinsky C, et. al. Changes in Burnout and Satisfaction with Work-Life Integration in Physicians and the General US Working Population Between 2011 and 2017. Mayo Clinic Proceedings, February 22, 2019. doi: https://doi.org/10.1016.mayocp.2018.10.023.

3. Yasgur BS, Challenging Stigma: Should Psychiatrists Disclose Their Own Mental Illness? *Psychiatry Advisor*, January 11, 2019.

4. Gold KJ, Andrew LB, Goldman E, Schwenk TL. "I Would Never Want To Have a Mental Health Diagnosis on My Record": A Survey of Female Physicians on Mental Health Diagnosis, Treatment, and Reporting. *Gen Hosp Psychiatry.* 2016;43:51-57.

5. Holohan M. 'Silver Lining' of 2020: Medical and Nursing Schools See Increase in Applications. Today.com, December 22, 2020.

6. Llaurant M, van der Biezen M, Wijers N, Watananirun IK, Kontopantelis E, van Vught AJ. Nurses as Substitutes for Doctors in Primary Care. *Cochrane Database Syst Rev.* 2018;7: CD001271.doi:10.1002/14651858.CD001271.pub3.

7. Primary Care Coalition. Compare the Education Gaps Between Primary Care Physicians and Nurse Practitioners. Texas Academy of Family Physicians website. Tafp.org/Media/Default/Downloads/advocacy/scope-education.pdf.

8. Sarzenski E, Barry H. Current Evidence and Controversies: Advanced Practice Providers in Healthcare. *Am J Manag Care.* 2019;25(8):366-368.

9. American Medical Association. Code of Ethics. ama-assn.org.

10. American Medical Association. Ama-assn.org.

11. Association of American Medical Colleges. Policy Priorities to Improve Out Nation's Health How Medical Education Is Changing. Association of American Medical Colleges. aamc.org.

12. Buja LM. Medical Education Today: All That Glitters Is Not Gold. BMC Med Educ. 2019;19(1):110.

13. Ludmerer K. *Time to Heal: American Medical Education From the Turn of the Century to the Era of Managed Care.* New York: Oxford University Press; 1999, p.313.

14. Humphrey H. Resources for Medical Education: Finding the Right Prescription. *Trans Am Clin Climatol Assoc.* 2010;121:76-90.

15. Bohmer R. Managing The New Primary Care: The New Skills That Will Be Needed. *Health Aff (Millwood).* 2010;29(5):1010-14.

16. Flexner, A. *Medical Education: A Comparative Study.* New York: Macmillan; 1925, p. 148.

17. Flexner A. *Medical Education in the United States and Canada.* New York: Sagawan Press; 2105, p.26.

18. Hlavinka E. Racial Bias in Flexner Report Permeates Medical Education Today— Landmark Study Forced All but Two Black U.S. Medical Schools to Close. *MedPage Today.* June 18, 2020.

19. Flexner A. Medical Education in the United States and Canada; A Report to the Carnegie Foundation for the Advancement of Teaching. New York:Carnegie Foundation for the Advancement of Teaching;1910 http://archive.carnegiefoundation.org/publications/pdfs/elibrary/Carnegie_Flexner_Report.pdf. p. 179.

20. Bailey M. The Flexner Report: Standardizing Medical Students Through Region-, Gender-, and Race-Based Hierarchies. *Am J Law Med.* 2017;43(2-3):209-23.

21. Flexner A. *Medical Education in the United States and Canada, 1910.* Republished in *The Classics of Medicine Library.* Bethesda, MD: Gryphon Editions; 1990, p. 48.

22. Ludmerer, pp. 301, 309, 358-361.

23. Dyrbye LN, Thomas MR, Shanafelt TD. Medical Student Distress: Causes, Consequences, and Proposed Solutions. *Mayo Clin Proc.* 2005;80(12):1613-22.

24. Hill K A, Samuels EA, Gross CP. Assessment of the Prevalence of Medical Student Mistreatment by Sex, Race/Ethnicity, and Sexual Orientation. *JAMA Internal Med.* 2020;180(5):653-65. 0

25. Ludmerer, p. 313.

26. Starr P. *The Social Transformation of American Medicine.* New York, NY: Harper Collins;1982, p. 356.

27. Colwill J, Cultice J, Kruse R. Will Generalist Physician Supply Meet Demands of an Increasing and Aging Population? *Health Aff (Millwood),* 2008; 27(3):w232-w241.

28. Council on Graduate Medical Education. *Physician Workforce Policy Guidelines for the United States, 2000-2020.* Sixteenth Report. January 2005. www.cogme.gov/16.pdf.

29. Porter M, Teisberg E. *Redefining Health Care. Creating Value-Based Competition on Results.* Boston: Harvard Business Press; 2006, p. 220.

30. Institute of Medicine, Committee on Behavioral and Social Sciences in Medical School Curricula. In: *Improving Medical Education: Enhancing the Behavioral and Social Science Content of Medical School Curricula.* Washington, DC: National Academies Press; 2004, pp. 4, 9-11.

31. American Medical Association. Accelerating Change in Medical Education: Innovations and Outcomes of the Consortium. Ama-assn.org.

32. Lahey T, Ogrinc G, Fall L, et al. The Compelling Need for Education Reform: A Futurist's View of Health Professions Education. In: *Transformation of Academic Health Centers, Meeting the Challenge of Healthcare's Changing Landscape.* Washington, DC: Association of Academic Health Centers; 2015; pp. 121-33.

33. Izzo J, Klein E. *Awakening Corporate Soul: Fourth Paths to Unleash the Power of People at Work.* Beverly, MA: Fairwinds Press; 1999, pp. 34-7.

34. Bohmer R. Managing the New Primary Care: The New Skills That Will be Needed. *Health Aff (Millwood).* 2010;29(5):1010-14.

35. Ziegenfuss JT Jr, Sassani JW. Health Administration Education for Physicians: Why? *Am J Med Qual.* 2008 Jan-Feb;23(1):5-6.

CHAPTER 5: WE STARTED AS HEROES

Leadership Implications and Health Policy Considerations

Leadership Implications:

1. Medical education reform is traditionally approached through the formal curriculum. Understand the informal curriculum transmuted by the training environment as a crucial in developing effective physician leaders.
2. Understand the traits common to those selected for medical school and evaluate what traits should be developed to create strong physician leaders impacting the field of health services management.

Health Policy Considerations:

1. Understand the needs for medical education policy reform to support the advancement of didactic and experiential learning models that strengthen skills in management, strategic thinking, teamwork, and communication.
2. Evaluate potential innovations in medical education arising from the American Rescue Plan Act of 2021.

PART II

The Future Is Ours to Make

The Pace of Change Accelerates

Health and health care are going digital. As multiple intersecting plat-forms evolve to form a novel operational foundation for health and health care — the nation's digital health utility — the stage is set for fundamental and unprecedented transformation.[1]

IOM Roundtable on Value & Science Driven Healthcare (2010)

Artificial intelligence could have more profound implications for humanity than electricity or fire.[2]

Sunder Pichai, CEO Alphabet at Google I/O Conference May 17, 2017

The 21st-century technological innovations in communication and knowledge management are transforming the United States health-care system, just as they are every other segment of American society. Amidst all the barriers and challenges to improvement in healthcare delivery, the adoption of new technologies and processes of information exchange are accelerating the pace of change in the delivery of health services, promising the possibility of a true renaissance in the way we live and work in our healthcare organizations.

Several innovations are enhancing physicians' ability to improve patient care by radically altering the processes and mechanisms through which health-care services may be delivered.

We are just beginning to fully embrace some of the advancements in com-munication that will strengthen the ability to improve the lives of patients. Many of the changes just over the horizon, such as artificial intelligence-enhanced clinical decision support, will be extraordinarily disruptive to the healthcare *status quo*, and much of the current healthcare delivery system is ill-prepared for the impact of the impending technological renaissance.

The critical areas where technological innovations have the greatest potential to improve care are:

- **Communication among patients, clinical teams, and stakeholders.** The traditional physician-patient relationship has tended to be focused on the face-to-face exchange of information in a healthcare facility setting. The incorporation of social media, personal health records, and health information exchange across the spectrum of settings of care changes both the temporal and spatial boundaries of communication of the doctor-patient relationship.
- **Improvement in quality and safety of healthcare services.** A reduction in medical errors is possible with the implementation of new tools with advanced predictive capabilities, including clinical decision support and artificial intelligence. Remote evaluation, diagnosis, and monitoring through telehealth technologies are pushing the boundaries of preventive and precision medicine out of the exam room into the patient's home and workplace, thereby bringing healthcare services directly to the patient rather than requiring the patient to present to the health services facility.

As these new technologies evolve and others emerge, the role of physicians will also change. Physicians who are committed to leading in the healthcare delivery system, such that patient care is improved within the realm of these rapid changes, may find it useful to understand the concepts behind complexity theory as it pertains to complex adaptive systems. Times of a highly accelerated pace of change may result in possibilities for great improvement, but also significant disruption in traditional systems of care.

The emergence of new innovations may or may not improve the quality of care in the complex adaptive system of healthcare. Careful attention by physician leaders to three important aspects of communication within the complex adaptive system may increase the likelihood that quality is improved. Physicians practicing in the new virtual dimensions of healthcare must understand patterns of relationships,[3] feedback processes, and assortativity.[4]

Social media's emerging role in physician communication with patients and clinical teams is creating new relationship patterns that were not part of the physician's role as little as 20 years ago. Combined with new capabilities in telehealth, health information exchange, and personal health records, new dimensions in communication will provide the potential ability to improve the quality of care.

The sheer speed and scale made possible by the exponentially faster information exchange engendered by quantum computing will create artificial-intelligence platforms capable of monitoring physiological responses in real-time and processing diagnostic possibilities with speed and precision heretofore impossible. The primary provider of healthcare information role previously held by clinical experts may no longer be an essential component of the physician-patient relationship.

The role of expertise will change when clinicians compete directly with quantum computers. Instead, through effective feedback processes, healthcare providers can mitigate ambiguity and ensure clarity in order for patients to understand better and actively participate in decisions impacting their care.

Within the discipline of complexity science, *assortativity* describes *nodes* within a *system*, their tendencies to connect to other nodes, and the number of connections of each node. Within the conceptual framework of a complex adaptive system, each physician, provider organization, and payer organization can be viewed as an individual node within a unique set of connection points to patients and to one another.

Technological innovation disrupts traditional nodal connections and creates new ones. Physician leaders who understand the application of the concept may be able to increase efficiency within the delivery of health services and patient care by developing more person-centered design processes.

Patient-centered care is also one of the IOM's six aims for improvement in healthcare. The *Crossing the Quality Chasm* report identifies the dimensions of patient-centered care as:[5]

• Respect for patients' values, preferences, and expressed needs.
• Coordination and integration of care.
• Information, communication, and education.
• Physical comfort.
• Emotional support-relieving fear and anxiety.
• Involvement of family and friends.

The underlying theme of the IOM report focuses on the difficulty in providing such patient-centered care in the current complex healthcare system. Notwithstanding such difficulty, successful integration of these new technologies may permit adaptation of the system in ways that enhance the goals of patient-centered care.

STRENGTHENING COMMUNICATION

The recognition that electronic health information exchange could strengthen communication and potentially improve patient outcomes came about early in the Information Age. President George W. Bush established the position of National Coordinator for Health Information Technology on April 27, 2004, through an executive order that Congress later mandated in the Health Information Technology for Economic and Clinical Health Act (HITECH) that was part of the American Recovery and Reinvestment Act of 2009.

Since its inception, the Office of the National Coordinator for Health Information Technology (ONC) has been focused on increasing end-user adoption of electronic health records and other health information technology, establishing standards so various technologies can exchange information, providing incentives for market-driven clinical advances, protecting personal health information through privacy and security, and creating governance and structure for health information exchange.

The ONC established programs to facilitate these goals, including the health information technology extension program, the state health information exchange cooperative agreement program, the strategic health information advanced research projects (SHARP) program, the Beacon Community Program, and several community college and university-based training programs. ONC programs include the development of a federal HIT strategic plan and the establishment of governance for the nationwide health information network.

Although many of these grant-funded initiatives have been completed, the ongoing work of the ONC remains focused on the two strategic objectives of advancing the development and use of health IT capabilities and establishing an expectation for data sharing.

The 21st Century Cures Act was signed into law on December 13, 2016, and updated some of the ONC's efforts by mandating the ONC establish a common framework to enable nationwide health information exchange. The 21st Century Cures Act established the funding for the development of the Trusted Exchange Network that will act as a large health information network that healthcare providers can use to easily share and exchange electronic records.

The second draft of the Trusted Exchange Framework and Common Agreement (TEFCA), released in 2019, sets forth a common set of principles designed to establish minimum required terms and conditions and technical standards for national health information exchange. Over the course of the next several years, these standards will serve as an interoperability roadmap that will permit coordinated health information exchange.

In 2021, the United States Qualified Health Information Network (USQHIN) was formed as a wholly owned subsidiary of Velatura Public Benefit Corporation, itself spun out of the Michigan Health Information Network in 2018. USQHIN has announced its intention to be a qualified health information network under TEFCA and sees itself as different from existing networks that are largely focused on connecting large EMR systems.[6]

USQHIN is currently working on a National ADT Hub Network to create a mechanism for exchanging admission, discharge, and transfer (ADT) data exchange to better enable national public health use cases and various federal interoperability goals. The pandemic has highlighted the inefficiencies inherent in the currently fragmented vendor and HIE model in the country, and efforts of USQHIN to provide a more efficient national solution are timely.

THE PERILS AND PROMISE OF PRECISION MEDICINE

For decades, the care delivery model has been based on an intuitive approach to the practice of medicine. But with these technological enablers comes a refinement in the culture of medicine such that the ability to deliver care that is more rigorous and precise will become standard. In *The Innovator's Prescription*, Christensen, Grossman, and Hwang note that:

> . . . progress along the spectrum between intuitive and precision medicine is the primary mechanism through which technological enablers can lead the disruption of existing healthcare business models.[7]

Technologically enabled scientific progress may enhance the art of medicine by adapting systems of care that can focus upon the IOM's patient-centered values. New diagnostic and testing technologies arising from advancements in pharmacogenomics are driving precision medicine such that healthcare can be much more individualized. Electronic health records, personal health records, clinical decision support tools, and other health information technologies will also contribute to the shift away from intuitive medicine and toward greater refinement of the industry's ability to diagnose and deliver care at the population level. The collaborative ingenuity and drive to deliver higher quality care by clinical teams will permit the nuances of incremental design and development of new innovations to improve care delivery rather than simply disrupt it.

Technology accelerates fundamental changes to the traditional healthcare business models. The provider-centered, facility-focused approach to care is giving way to patient-focused care models where technology empowers convenience, 24/7 access, and evidence-based standards that eliminate unwarranted variation. Patients become informed consumers participating in shared decisions. They are highly engaged, socially connected, and have healthcare access through mobile devices anytime.

With the advent of whole genomic sequencing, artificial intelligence, and CRISPR technologies, basic health management will yield to genome-linked life plans focused on monitoring and prevention. One-size-fits-all medicine will be replaced by personalized therapies, accurate diagnostics, and individualized, tailored pharmaceuticals. The business models that sustained the traditional healthcare ecosystem will no longer work. Blockbuster drugs that sustained the pharmaceutical industry in the past have very different pricing and financial models than precision cancer therapies.

Likewise, the healthcare payer methodologies built on actuarial risk projections have been based on population averages and trends in spending sets insurance prices. Predictive modeling and precision medicine destroy the payer system business model built on bell curves and markups.

Precision medicine holds enormous promise in transforming healthcare:

- **Precision medicine enables better diagnostics**.
  Diagnostic odysseys will diminish as idiopathic conditions will be mapped to specific genetic variances. Genome-wide association studies (GWAS) will improve the understanding of complex disease risk factors. More precise diagnostics can eliminate unnecessary testing and enhance patient safety.

- **Precision medicine improves therapeutics.**
  Recently, pharmacogenomics more accurately predict therapeutic response in patients with major depression and bipolar disease. Greatly improved adherence for patients with schizophrenia with companion diagnostic tests screening for side effects has been demonstrated. Targeted cancer drugs are improving long-term survival in metastatic disease.

- **Precision medicine creates better approaches to prevention**.
  The convergence of biology and information will shift traditional health system approaches from reactive to proactive healthcare. Early personalized interventions can integrate with population surveillance to enable robust, complex clinical decision support. Predictive modeling with open, dynamic knowledge banks can create a democratized health information commons.

Predictably, the healthcare industry's response has been slow to recognize the implications of these changes. Challenges to the uptake and integration

Our healthcare quality improvement methodologies are based upon 19th-century Gaussian mathematics.

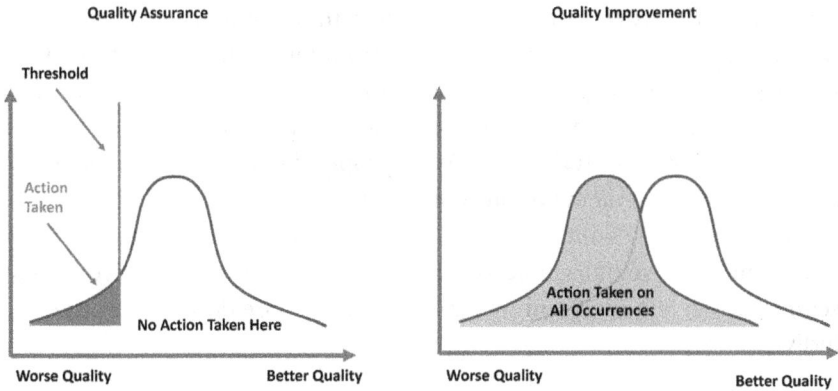

Figure 1.

of personalized medicine in clinical practice include barriers related to value demonstration. There is a lack of education and awareness among patients and healthcare professionals and a lack of patient empowerment with respect to access to precision medicine tools.

The lack of value recognition from the payer industry, both clinical and economic, is problematic. Precision medicine is not focused on large randomized controlled clinical trials by its very nature. The uncertainty of evidence requirement for coverage and reimbursement creates an access hurdle. The lack of effective healthcare delivery infrastructure and information management systems to use personalized medicine exists where resources are focused on traditional electronic health records rather than predictive modeling technologies.

However, every practicing physician knows that every single day we see patients that just don't fit into neatly stratified categories. This recognition is the quintessential component of medical practice and the use of precision technology can get us back to our roots of making sure the patient in front of us is getting the best possible care for them, not for an imaginary "average" patient.

From this patient-centered perspective, precision medicine may move the healthcare system from its singular focus on eliminating *unwarranted* variation to a refocus on *warranted* variation. The recent emphasis of the Institute of Medicine (IOM) on improving the diagnostic process is the right direction.

The IOM's goals of improving diagnosis and reducing diagnostic error emphasize the need to establish work systems and culture that support the diagnostic process and improvements in diagnostic performance as well as a payment and care delivery environment that supports the diagnostic process. Appropriate integration of genetic testing and other precision medicine technologies into the diagnostic process will accelerate the achievement of these IOM goals. With proper design, precision technologies can return medicine to our core mission. It is a tailored approach to healthcare that accounts for individual variability in the genes, environment, and lifestyle of each person that may lead to more effective patient segmentation and interventions and systems of care designed around the individual patient.

Physicians have the opportunity to lead the healthcare delivery system to a better understanding of the intersection of precision medicine and population health and the need for business models that will support this intersection. Value-based care is focused on shared savings and risk payments and are organized around populations, conditions, and efficient care delivery. Precision medicine can improve population health by moving the value drivers from efficiency not just at the population level, but at the individual patient level.

Rather than emphasizing the quality process measures inherent in the current delivery system, the N of 1 analytic modeling in precision medicine can permit quality measures designed around outcomes. Information management and patient differentiation capabilities can drive profit pools and new business models built on information integration predictive analytics and whole-person focused design.

The capabilities inherent in 21st-century technology will substantially disrupt the healthcare ecosystems built on older analytic methods. The convergence of biology and information and the economic imperatives of system change will disrupt business models to shift from reactive to proactive healthcare constructed on precision pathways, personalization, and prediction designed with complex clinical decision support, statistical thinking, dynamic modelling, knowledge banks and data mining, workflow-embedded practice guidelines, and pay-for-success business models.

Core clinical strategies can be formed from the identification of patient variation built into clinical workflows, a focus on analytics to increase the diagnostic rate to drive the development of more effective clinical models, and integration into effective models of care to drive therapeutic development.

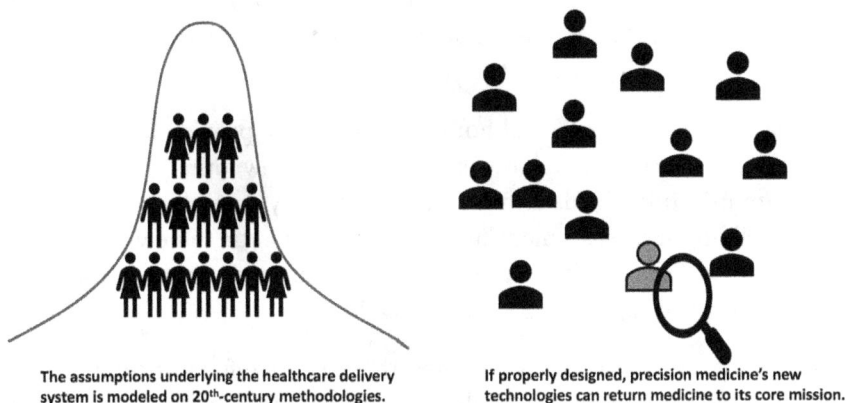

The assumptions underlying the healthcare delivery system is modeled on 20th-century methodologies.

If properly designed, precision medicine's new technologies can return medicine to its core mission.

Figure 2.

Precision medicine will integrate behavioral, clinical, and social risk into models of care that provide superior value. However, the variability in Internet access across the population as demonstrated during the pandemic needs to be addressed upfront. Disruptive innovation subsumes important challenges yet to be addressed.

First, the reimbursement models are ill-defined. As the industry moves toward performance-based accountable models of care, ensuring that compensation strategies are in place, putting these tools to use in patient care practices will be crucial to the success of these initiatives.

Second, variation in patients' access to electronic tools, particularly those in the underserved, impoverished, rural, and elderly populations, makes systematic use of such individualized tools fragmented at best. Physician leadership needs to address these challenges within the context of equitable and efficient care. The frontline experience of physicians providing care to patients will be necessary in the extraordinary potential for these disruptive innovations both to enhance and hinder effective care.

IMPLICATIONS OF SOCIAL TECHNOLOGY FOR THE THERAPEUTIC RELATIONSHIP

Patterns of Relationships. Kurtz and Snowden studied the impact of the inherent variability in interactions in human behavior and communication.[8] Their focus on the need to understand patterns of relationships may help improve doctor-patient communication by deconstructing the impact of new forms of electronic media on patterns of communication.

Electronic communication applications provide new structural support that enables the formation of relationships where they were not previously possible.

The patient-centered medical home is intended to provide for improved coordination of care through the enhancement of new forms and structures of communication. Fields and colleagues[9] identify several elements critical to building successful medical home models that tie to new patterns of relationships, including the development of dedicated non-physician care coordinators and expanded access to providers.

The Affordable Care Act established the objective for putting in place interdisciplinary community health teams to support the implementation of medical homes. New communication processes need to be established in patient relations to improve coordination which will in turn lead to the unfolding of new patterns in relationships and drive the evolution of clinical workflow processes. Improving access also means growing relationships by creating new opportunities for electronic communication between physicians and their patients.

Variation in cultural expectations of relationships is inherent in differences in technological capacities, geographic locations, and generational norms. The impact of chronic disease and illness specific to the elderly must be considered when evaluating patterns of relationships and the community impact of changes generated by healthcare reform. Physician leadership in understanding these relational patterns is important to ensure that workflows and processes of physician practices and integrated health systems are congruent with established patterns and needs of patients in the relationships they maintain with them. The ability to manage relationships effectively and understand them within the greater context of community obligation is part of the duty to society and professional obligation to the patients served.

Feedback Processes. New patterns of feedback embedded in health information technology have the potential to impact health outcomes in entirely unexpected ways. The critical processes by which people receive feedback, enhancing decision-making abilities, are used to react to changes in the environment. In turn, the information received can alter an individual's course of action and thus generate change in the system as a whole.

Information received may be positive or negative and can affect change within the individual or system. For example, a patient may ask a question of a physician through a mobile application, patient portal, or some other digital front door, or they may post a question to an online social network regarding the same issue. They receive one response (or feedback) from the physician but could receive multiple responses through other channels. The ensuing actions taken by the patient are put in motion to a greater or lesser extent based on the feedback received.

One of the challenges lies in improving patient adherence to evidence-based therapy and understanding what forms of feedback have the greatest impact. Any feedback received varies in degrees of clarity, ambiguity, and accuracy. The ability of the recipient to distill the applicability, validity, and value of the information received and to determine an appropriate course of action will directly affect the patient's health outcomes.

Healthcare workers who experience "alert fatigue" from an overabundance of alarms embedded in electronic devices such as monitors, computerized order entry programs, and electronic health records in the healthcare environment may experience unsuccessful outcomes from clinical support tools due to inappropriate, poorly engineered forms of feedback.

Associativity. Online social networks developed for healthcare purposes have metamorphosized the nature of health information exchange. Electronic communities such as *PatientsLikeMe* have rapidly grown in their importance for increasing connectivity among patients experiencing common illnesses and diseases.[10]

The expanse of social media platforms and portals that have emerged is extensive and includes a vast array of options for consumers and physicians alike. Tools such as Microsoft Health Vault, WebMD, and Up-to-Date are examples of new electronic applications that have broken down boundaries that once limited access to timely health information.

In the web-based dimension of society that has evolved, patients and their physicians have become more apt to cross these boundaries and make connections that can lead to improvement in quality of care. Patients may learn from one another about important aspects of their medical condition directly from peer-to-peer web-based patient communities that do not involve the expertise of professional healthcare providers at all. Likewise, there are opportunities for physicians to communicate, collaborate, and exchange ideas in secured online "physician-only" communities such as Doximity, Sermo, DailyRounds, and QuantiaMD, which are doctor-focused social networking sites offering connection, crowd-sourcing, and education opportunities.

Associativity characterizes the degree of interconnectedness between various nodes within a system. As noted by Foster and colleagues, online social networks tend to exhibit traits of both associativity and disassociativity, such that networks focused on driving patient-to-patient communication have the ability to improve patient knowledge and amass data for use within the medical community.

In these types of networks, each node (e.g., a patient) can have a multitude of connections and will be limited in their degree of connectedness only based on privacy and security levels established for their profiles and communication conducted within the network. This degree of potential associativity can translate into opportunities for many connections to each node and a low chance of failure to make desired connections within the online community.

Networks that focus on physician-to-physician communications have the potential for greater reward/loss because of the value and sensitivity of information shared and its potential to directly improve patient care. However, typically there are fewer "qualified" connections that can influence clinical and business decision-making in these scenarios due to their exclusivity.

Physician peer networks increase opportunities to engage in and drive communication across new mediums and channels that have the potential to save time, reduce the cost of care, and extend efforts to make use of evidence-based medicine practices. Peer-to-peer communication among physicians may provide invaluable opportunities to share best practices and clinical knowledge to improve abilities to deliver optimal care beyond geographic markets.

New opportunities exist for the physician community to use electronic media to engage across multiple interconnected dimensions of communication in their daily work: physician to patient, physician to physician, physician to vendor, physician to payer, physician to caregiver, physician to community resource center, physician to clinical care team, and physician to pharmacy.

Highly important for physician leaders are those forms of communication that connect them to vendors, third-party payers, government regulators, employers, and other healthcare stakeholders who are not directly involved in patient care. Management and oversight of communication with vendors are critical in light of Federal Trade Commission monitoring and medicolegal issues involving relations with pharmaceutical companies and medical device companies.

Accurate and timely information exchange is essential for efficient management of the revenue cycle, auditing and coding requirements, and required public reporting. Enhanced efforts to diminish fraud have resulted in programs such as the CMS Recovery Audit Contractor Program.

In summary, management in the complex adaptive system that constitutes the healthcare delivery system may be understood by analyzing change in the system through the patterns of relationships, feedback processes, and associativity of various parts of the system. Through these filtering lenses, we may achieve greater insight and, therefore an ability to lead by managing these complex variables.

IMPROVING QUALITY AND SAFETY

The history of the development of health information technology demonstrates that the technology has tended to focus first on the business aspects of medicine; secondarily on the clinical aspects; and, only recently, to advance population management.

For at least 30 years, sophisticated practice management systems have been available for purposes of billing and collections, coding and auditing, claims management, and scheduling based upon a delivery system focused on episodic care. Over the past 20 years, electronic health records have been developed that are far from mature products in terms of the ultimate goal of sophisticated improvement in clinical care, and population management information infrastructure is in its infancy.

Much of the electronic health records in use today have been designed for maximizing fee-for-service billing documentation rather than efficient clinical workflow. In a study published just prior to the pandemic, a cross-sectional survey of U.S. physicians from all specialty disciplines concluded the usability of current EHR systems received a grade of F by physician users when evaluated using a standardized metric of technology usability. The study also observed a strong dose-response relationship between EHR usability and the odds of burnout.[11]

In response to the study, the American Medical Association Advisory Committee on EHR Physician Usability issued a white paper in which they identified key challenges physicians face with current EHRs:[10]

- Interference with the patient visit.
- Lack of system-design support for team-based care.
- Issues with care coordination due to lack of interoperability.
- Increased cognitive workload for physicians.
- Lack of data liquidity and high switching costs.

- Lack of product modularity to support unique physician practices and population needs.
- Communicating with patients in a changing digital landscape.
- Insufficient support for incorporating end-user input into product design and post-implementation feedback for product improvement.

The task force also delineated eight EHR usability priorities around which the AMA intends to work with vendors, advocate for federal and state policymakers, collaborate with healthcare systems to develop effective institutional health IT policies, and educate physicians about these priorities:

- Enhance physicians' ability to provide high-quality patient care.
- Support team-based care.
- Promote care coordination.
- Offer product modularity and configurability.
- Reduce cognitive workload
- Promote data liquidity
- Facilitate digital and mobile patient engagement
- Expedite user input into product design and post-implementation feedback. [12]

To improve healthcare quality, physician leaders need to embrace the development of electronic health records designed for usability and work with the vendor and regulatory communities to guide appropriate care management applications of population management information infrastructure. Physicians will need to lead organizations in several areas in this regard, including security and accessibility of information, clinical workflow, and advanced health information technology systems.

Security and Accessibility of Information. The security of patient health information has become a growing concern in the age of the digitization of all patient medical records. Electronic health records raise the prevalence of threats of breaches of information security and unlawful access to patient health information.

HIPAA regulations were strengthened substantially with the passage of the HITECH Act, resulting in stronger civil and criminal penalties for those who engage in such acts, and enforcement was extended to include "covered entities" or business associates of healthcare organizations. Cases of security breaches occur across the spectrum of healthcare stakeholder organizations, including integrated health systems, insurance payer organizations (public and private), academic medical centers, physician practice groups, and reference labs. The causes of these breaches have varied, including design flaws in technology permitting unintentional human error and/or willful misconduct on behalf of personnel who have access to such information.

Expanded use of data encryption and requirements for digital signatures for secure messages that include patient health information and improved authentication and authorization methods will strengthen the national health information technology infrastructure.[13] Physician leadership that embraces the patient's right to privacy within the traditional bounds of the doctor-patient relationship and in the new relational, associative world of electronic interconnectivity will go a long way toward strengthening the trust of patients and the general public in the healthcare community's ability to protect their personal health information.

Clinical Workflow. The redesign implications for integrating new technology solutions into the daily workflow of clinicians is an essential element in improving the quality and safety of healthcare services in primary care and tertiary care settings. In 2008, the Joint Commission issued Sentinel Report #42, which identified a number of actions for organizations to take to reduce the risk of medical errors that result from health information technology implementations:[14]

> Examine workflow processes and procedures for risks and inefficiencies and resolve these issues prior to any technology implementation. Involving representatives of all disciplines — whether they be clinical, clerical or technical — will help in the examination and resolution of these issues.

The flow of clinical work processes through every physician practice, clinic, skilled nursing facility, house call, or hospital organization represents all the procedures and activities, ranging from simple to complex, required to deliver patient care services within these settings. Multidisciplinary teams must engage from across an organization to effectively analyze current processes and determine the redesign of future clinical processes for patient care.

As the industry continues the move toward models of clinical integration and accountable care, there is an increasingly greater need for physician involvement in collaboration with multidisciplinary partners to map out new clinical workflows that reduce waste and potential for medical errors that occur in care delivery settings, ranging from treatment plan creation and management to disease/condition diagnosis, medication prescribing, patient education, and procedure ordering.[15]

Standardized order sets can reduce variation and decrease errors and costs in electronic health records. But these benefits can stand in direct conflict with personalized, individualized patient-centered care. Physician leadership in the implementation process can mitigate this conflict such that patient-centeredness is not sacrificed for the sake of efficiency.

Though much of their work is becoming inherently more collaborative and team-based, physicians remain ultimately accountable for the care delivered to their patients. For this reason, physician leadership and engagement are essential in efforts to redefine and transform clinical workflow in healthcare organizations.

Advanced Health Information Technology Systems. Clinical decision support (CDS) and telemedicine tools for physicians are two key innovations that hold great promise for the future and have already made a significant impact on patient care capabilities. While the impact can be identified at individual patient case levels on a macro level, there is great application and meaning to physician leaders, especially with the adoption of telemedicine tools to help achieve broader community health objectives.

CDS involves the use of technologies that bring intelligent aids to the benefit of physicians and clinical/ancillary staff to help improve decision-making on issues related to patient care. CDS can be viewed as a knowledge-based and algorithm-driven tool that seeks to meet the challenges of complexity in decision making and automate the processes that historically have been used by physicians and other clinicians.

Artificial intelligence-based technology has been used effectively in other industries, such as the aerospace and defense sectors, for developing unattended ground and aerial vehicles as well as modeling and simulation tools. However, these engineering advances have only begun making their way into the development of clinical decision support in healthcare.

CDS tools can be divided into at least three categories: alerting CDS, workflow CDS, and cognitive CDS. Examples of *alerting* CDS are safety alerts issued for drug-to-drug interactions and sepsis alerts that provide early detection of problems developing with patients in the inpatient setting. *Workflow* CDS streamlines documentation requirements through use of standardized order sets. With a well-designed workflow, clinical decision support reduces the amount of manual data entry by physicians and their clinical teams. The third category, *cognitive* CDS, establishes point-of-service capabilities in evidence-based medicine to support physician clinical decisions.[16]

At the onset of the pandemic, the Center for Medicare and Medicaid Services (CMS) broadened access to Medicare telehealth by using a 1135 waiver such that for the first time, Medicare can pay for office, hospital, and other

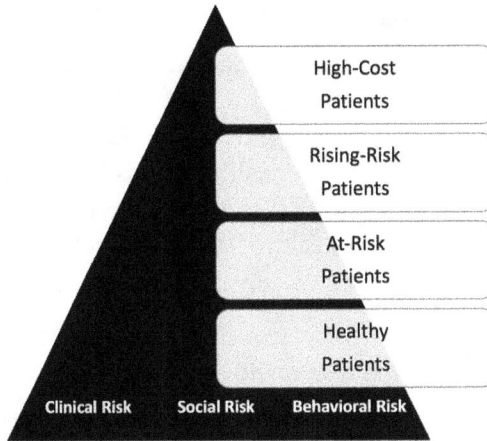

Whole-person care integrates behavioral, clinical, and social risk into models of care that provide superior value.

Figure 3.

visits furnished via telehealth. Initially effective on March 6, 2020, CMS has extended and clarified details of the waiver, which remains in place while the emergency declaration is in place.

The Telehealth Modernization Bill is before Congress to give the Health and Human Services Secretary the authority to permanently expand the types of telehealth services covered by Medicare and the types of care providers eligible to deliver these services. As a result of the Medicare expansion and similar policy changes by private payers, the use of telehealth services rose 2980% in 2020 compared to the previous year.[17]

Unfortunately, even as telehealth use rises, a digital divide exists based on the level of income. The expansion of telemedicine capabilities is the cornerstone technology of the Minnesota Beacon Community project. Physicians in rural areas have struggled with the lack of broadband access in their communities and with the high capital cost required to implement such tools. The 2009 ARRA and HITECH Act provide significant industry-level funding and support for improving the broadband access capabilities of the health information technology infrastructure throughout the country.

These investments in infrastructure development lower barriers to accessing these technologies, which require high-speed transmission of data such as telemedicine, electronic medical records, and health analytics systems. If well-designed, these initiatives will improve the quality of patient care, reduce medical errors, and eliminate redundant ordering.

REFLECTION POINTS

Federal funding and policy are driving the healthcare industry to use innovative technological solutions to mitigate many of its current challenges. The requirements of the CMS Meaningful Use for Electronic Health Records Program pushed physicians and health systems to implement electronic health records that met the federal certification criteria but were not necessarily built for efficient clinical workflow or effective population health management.

However, the need for more effective clinical decision support tools at the point of service, improved diagnostic capabilities through artificial intelligence, and precision medicine technologies will continue to transform the medical profession. Physician leaders who work to craft strategy, care for patients, and ensure that improvement in the quality of services is measurable will reestablish their traditional healer role in a modern, population-focused context.

In 2010, the IOM and ONC-HIT convened the Roundtable for Value & Science Driven Healthcare. The focus of the roundtable was to bring together a group of industry experts through a series of workshops to assess the state of the industry and the "digital health utility." The group acknowledged challenges faced by the healthcare industry due to its complexity. A key theme for their effort was that:

> . . . transformative influences of information technology on society over the past three decades is a blended product of interrelated initiatives arising from within the commercial, independent, and public sectors.19

A convergence of interests across these sectors and across competing clusters has resulted in a politicized dialogue regarding the healthcare industry's future path. Physicians must rise to the challenge of leading organizations through this period of technological and cultural transformation that is certain to accelerate. Their willingness to support the expansion and utility of technological innovation is a crucial step to improving the quality of care and measurable health outcomes. The achievement of greater balance and distribution of resources in the U.S. healthcare system by leveraging advances in technology and communication may improve our ability to provide the right care at the right time.

REFERENCES

1. Yong PL, Olsen la, McGinnis JM. Institute of Medicine (US) Roundtable on Value & Science-Driven Health Care. Washington, DC: National Academices Press (US); 2010.

2. Cuthbertson A. What's Bigger Than Fire and Electricity? Artificial Intelligence, Says Google Boss. Newsweek. January 22, 2018.

3. *Learning About Complexity Science.* NAPCRG Resources. August 2009.

4. Foster J, Foster D, Grassberger P, Paczuski M. Edge Direction and the Structure of Networks. *PNAS.* 2010;107(24):10815-20.

5. Institute of Medicine, Committee on Quality of Health Care in America. *Crossing the Quality Chasm.* Washington, DC: National Academies Press; 2006, pp. 49-50.

6. Leventhal R. United States QHIN Established as 'Alternative Health Information Network.' Healthcare Innovation. February 8, 2021. www.hcinnovationgroup. com/interoperability-hie/trusted-exchange-framework-and-common-agreement-tefca/news/21209250/united-states-qhin-established-as-alternative-health-information-network

7. Christensen C, Grossman J, Hwang J. *The Innovator's Prescription: A Disruptive Solution for Health Care.* New York, NY: McGraw-Hill;2009, p. 45.

8. Kurtz CF, Snowden DJ. The New Dynamics of Strategy: Sense-making in a Complex and Complicated World. *IBM Systems Journal.* 2003;42(3):462-83.

9. Fields D, Leshen E, Kavita P. Driving Quality Gains and Cost Savings Through Adoption of Medical Homes. *Health Aff (Millwood)* 2010;29(5)819-26.

10. Christensen C, Grossman J, Hwang J. *The Innovator's Prescription: A Disruptive Solution for Health Care.* New York, NY: McGraw-Hill; 2009, pp. 24-25.

11. Melnci E, Dyrbye L, Sinsky C, Nedeled L, Tutty M, Shanafelt T. The Association Between Perceived Electronic Health Record Usability and Professional Burnout Among US Physicians. *Mayo Clinic Proceedings.* 2020;95(3):P476-87. March 1, 2020.

12. American Medical Association. Improving Care: Priorities to Improve Electronic Health Record Usability. AMA;2104. www.ama-assn.org/sites/ama-assn.org/files/corp/media-browser/member/about-ama/ehr-priorities.pdf

13. President's Council of Advisors on Science and Technology. *Report to the President. Realizing The Full Potential of Health Information Technology To Improve Healthcare For Americans: The Path Forward.* 2010. Chapter V. Privacy & Security. pp. 45-52.

14. The Joint Commission. Sentinel Event Alert 42: Implementing Health Information and Converging Technologies. 2008 Dec 11;(42):1-4.

15. Bowens FM, Frye PA, Jones WA. Health Information Technology: Integration of Clinical Workflow into Meaningful Use of Electronic Health Records. *Perspect Health Inf Manag.* 2010 Fall; 7(Fall): 1d.

16. Richardson J, Ash J, Sittig D, Bunce A, Carpenter J, et. al. Multiple Perspectives on the Meaning of Clinical Decision Support. *AMIA Annu Symp Proc.* 2010; 2010:1427-31.

17. Gelburd R. Telehealth Claim Lines Rise 2980% in One-Year Period Through September 2020. AJMC. December 1, 2020. www.ajmc.com/view/telehealth-claim-lines-rise-2980-in-one-year-period-through-september-2020

CHAPTER 6: THE PACE OF CHANGE ACCELERATED
Leadership Implications and Health Policy Considerations

Leadership Implications:

1. Understand the potential impact of precision medicine on health care services delivery and how the physician-patient role may change.
2. Analyze the technological innovations under development that may advance new opportunities to improve access and quality of care.

Health Policy Considerations:

1. Stay abreast of federal and state policy reforms in the health information technology domain including the 21st-Century Cures Act with its new requirements in health information exchange.
2. Physician leadership can focus federal and regional health information technology workgroups on the impact of health policy changes on complex adaptive systems.

Professionalism Is Redemption

What is likely to be most at risk for the professions is their freedom to set their own agenda for the development of their discipline and to assume responsibility for its use. Thus, the most important problem for the future of professionalism is neither economic nor structural but cultural and ideological. The most important problem is its soul.[1]

Eliot Freidson

Medicine and the other traditional professions developed in a world in which access to specialized knowledge was not readily available to most people. The special skills required to treat disease are developed through a prolonged medical education and presume that such work is "so specialized as to be inaccessible to those lacking the required training and experience, and . . . cannot be standardized, rationalized, or commodified."[2]

Such professions have unique control over their own work and thus are afforded a considerable degree of power and privilege. Consequently, holders of such specialized knowledge have specific obligations to those whom they serve due to the unequal relationship in power.

Much of the medical literature prior to the late 20th century that addressed the conceptual requirements of professionalism, therefore, emphasized the "right" behaviors by physicians in their interactions with their patients. In his essays on the physician-patient relationship in 1888, for example, S. Weir Mitchell, MD, LLD, stated that:

> The physician cannot be a mere intellectual machine. None know that better than we. Through all ages, we have insisted that he shall feel himself bound by a code of moral law, to which, on the whole, he has held without questions, while creeds of more serious nature were shifting and changing.[3]

Weir focused on *privacy* ("He must guard the secrets wrung from you on the rack of disease."), *empathy* ("The capacity to enter into, to realize, and hence to feel with and for you."), *objectivity* ("I once saw a very young physician who burst into tears at the sight of a burnt child, a charming young girl. He was practically useless for a time."), and *truthfulness* ("One is troubled to do what is right and to say in answer to their questions what is true.") as qualities of the physician's professionalism.[4] He believed that the physician must be one who is "competent, clear-headed, honest, scrupulously careful" but not "plain, ill-dressed, and uninteresting."[5]

By the late 20th century, the emphasis on specific types of professional behavior was codified in standards of professional ethics that focused on the responsibilities of the physician:

> . . . diagnosing the patient's condition, informing and educating the patient about his condition, including its prognosis if treated or untreated and about the various possible treatment alternatives, recommending the course of action that the physician considers the best medical approach for that individual's problems, and, carrying out those procedures, for example, monitoring, prescribing-that are required by the approach chosen for the patient.[6]

These specific behavioral responsibilities are integrated into the basic precepts of moral theory embedded in the values of *autonomy, nonmaleficence, beneficence,* and *justice* such that veracity, privacy, confidentiality, and fidelity are used as standards for defining appropriate clinical behavior.[7]

Beauchamp and Childress's work in biomedical ethics in the 1980s and 1990s sought to "move beyond principles, rules, obligations, and rights" and into a framework based on "virtues, ideals, and aspirations for moral excellence"[8] based on *compassion, discernment, integrity,* and *conscientiousness* "such that an Aristotelian framework in which innate human virtues are developed by appropriate training and exercise."[9]

They specifically discussed virtues and ideals in professional life within the metaphors of saints and heroes and cite four conditions[10] of moral excellence that must be met to achieve this heroic professional status:

+ "Faithfulness to a worthy moral ideal."
+ "A motivational structure conforming to patterns of virtuous persons."
+ "An exceptional moral character."
+ "Deep personal integrity."

These constructs of medical professionalism, defined within the context of moral behaviors obligated by the power invested in the authority of specialized knowledge, are in direct conflict with the rise of *managerialism* in the 20th century, which is based on "the authority to command, organize, guide, and supervise both the choices of consumers and the productive work of specialists."[11] Managers have power by virtue of their authority to allocate resources necessary for work.[12]

The rise of complex organizational infrastructure in the 20th century is the result of the invention of management in which claims of general knowledge that is "superior to specialization because it can organize it rationally and efficiently and falls back on its own special kind of preparation for positions of leadership — an advanced but general formal education that equips them to direct or lead specialists, consumers, and citizens."[13] Thus the "ideology of professionalism, which is generally rooted in specialization, contends with the challenge of populist generalism advanced by consumerism and elite generalism advanced by managerialism."[14]

As complex organizations rose in the 20th-century medical industry, the necessity of managerialism created a direct challenge to the traditional power and authority implicit in the old definitions of professionalism. The authority of the medical profession became relegated to the limited arena of their field of specialized knowledge. Rather than serving as an autonomous institution granting professional control over their work, the specialized knowledge was to "serve rather than command in the market and polity."[15]

As Freidson's "ideology of professionalism" indicated, a concern that the traditional professions were undergoing a process of "deprofessionalization" manifested by the late 20th century. The democratization of information by the Internet further challenged traditional views of professional authority. The tension between the authority granted professionals due to their expertise with the populist denial of any authority to specialized knowledge "literally deprofessionalized the labor force, the labor markets, and the organization of work."[16]

Many have claimed the professional status of medicine is weakening due to the access to medical information now available to the public through the Internet. Claims of authority based on specialized expertise alone do not permit adequate rationalization for authority if *expertise* is not seen as a quality separate from *information*.

The ideology of managerialism that denies authority to expertise by claiming its form of general knowledge is superior to specialized knowledge for allocation and organization of resources cannot in and of itself challenge professionalism without excluding the additional claim on the part of professionals that expertise must be coupled with specific forms of expected behavior. Thus, many of the recent approaches to medical professionalism have rediscovered the traditional focus on moral virtues and behaviors and sought to redefine professionalism within new social roles.

The American Medical Association (AMA) code of ethics from 1957 to 1980 urged physicians to be "upright" and "pure in character and diligent and conscientious in caring for the sick."[17] From 1980 to 2000, the AMA's code of ethics deemphasized virtues except for the admonition to "expose those physicians deficient in character or competence."[18] However, by 2001, the AMA refocused on moral virtue within the context of social responsibility.

In December 2001, the American Medical Association (AMA) issued its Declaration of Professional Responsibility.[19] In this declaration, physicians' duties are aligned with their global commitment as:

- Healers of the sick.
- Protectors of patient privacy and confidentiality.
- Drivers to work toward advances in medicine.
- Supporters of initiatives for the education and advocacy of change that improves the health and wellbeing of humanity.

In 2015, the *Journal of the American Medical Association (JAMA)* took a deep dive into professionalism, in one article emphasizing the responsibility and accountability of medicine to self-govern and self-regulate[20] and the ability to enhance professionalism through management skills in another.[21] Both points of view focused on how medical professionalism requires an updated approach to professionalism that keeps pace with the changing environment in which physicians practice:

> The leveling effect of social media and the Internet have changed the way citizens relate to each other and to their institutions, demanding a much more participatory and engaged style of leadership and more shared models of authority . . . physicians are continuously connected, embedded in teams, and reliant on technology and many other individuals to meet the needs of patients. Physicians confront previously unrecognized issues, like safety, shared decision making, and the expectation that physicians need to be involved-continuously-in making care better.[22]

> How should medical education be changed to enhance professionalism? One possible way is to incorporate systematic business and management education in medical school. . . . For physicians to improve their organizations' ability to reduce errors, improve patient safety, recognize and improve quality of care, incorporate new knowledge, ensure equitable care, reduce waste, and facilitate provision of services based on patients' values and interests, physicians need better management skills.[23]

The ideology of management, with its historical grounding in the development of complex organizations in the business community, is focused on planning, organizing, directing, controlling, monitoring, and decisional roles within companies.

Although social responsibility and ethics are discussed within management theory, the ethical emphasis tends to be on effectiveness and efficiency that make up much of the value system of capitalistic business models rather than personal and ethical responsibilities traditionally embodied in relationships between physicians and patients. So while the healthcare delivery system is most frequently organized into institutions with specific missions, visions, and values pertinent to the care of patients, the utilitarian approach to ethics that pervades business and organizational culture is substantially and qualitatively different from the individual relationship-based traditional and ethical approaches in medical professionalism.

However, the juxtaposition of the contrasting ideologies of managerialism and professionalism in the contemporary healthcare delivery system creates the opportunity for medical professionalism to be redefined not simply by areas of specialized medical expertise but also by unique, expected forms of behavioral and personal responsibility focused on service to patients.

The self-regulation of behavior that is intrinsic in the traditional autonomy granted to professions is as critical to maintaining status as a profession for physicians in the 21st century as it has historically been, and it must be focused on keeping patients safe, practicing high-quality care, and promoting health policies that are in the public interest.

An overemphasis by specialty societies and organized medicine in the financial and social wellbeing of physicians will lead to the public seeing physicians as one more special interest group looking out for itself and will lead to deprofessionalization of medicine as the public reacts with regulatory and market-based responses to perceived grievances. Thus, physicians must frame their claims to professional status not only in technical expertise but also codes of behaviors based on stewardship, servant leadership, and patient-centered approaches to policy advocacy.

Physician professional status is threatened when the caregiver aspects of the healer role are not incorporated into the overall cultural role. Sociologically, underemphasizing care-giving permits others to fill that important responsibility:

> Thus, American medicine, which has increasingly relied on the culture's male values of heroism and efficacy to legitimate its interventionalist

healthcare, has faced serious challenges from competitors justifying their own presence in the healthcare field with the female values of nurturance and forethought.[24]

Leicht and Fennell argue that the work that managers and professionals do is starting to look more similar due to changes in professional work brought on by the exponential growth in concerns about the accountability and prerogatives exercised by professionals resulting in external regulatory controls disrupting traditional professional routines.[25]

The perception of managers that they are entitled to control certain areas by virtue of their own judgments as managers led to a crisis of accountability on the part of medical professionals that is creating a convergence in the roles of professional and manager as physicians reacquaint themselves with the need for accountability within their professional role.

However, as physicians are increasingly employed by organizations where traditional sources of professional power are constrained, there is also a tendency for the development of stratification within the profession.[26]

In such complex organizational environments, the need to understand the general constructs that unify medicine as a profession must be understood within the diverse roles in which physicians practice.

Expertise and organizational role will deprofessionalize medicine without a commonly accepted understanding of expected behaviors, virtues, and values that are self-regulated, universal, and socially relevant regardless of institutional context.

This existentialist approach to medical professionalism provides a basis for leadership and differentiates the professional role of the physician from those aspects that are increasingly convergent with management or technical content experts, such as can be found in vocational fields such as engineering or airline piloting.

COMPETING CLUSTERS AND THE PHYSICIAN LEADER

The way healthcare is provided in the future may be markedly different from the way it is provided today, as information infrastructure and resource constraints move healthcare out of facilities and into homes and workplaces.

The enormous investment in capital resources in large hospital systems cannot continue to accelerate at its current pace. The boundaries of the healthcare delivery system will be redefined radically and rapidly. For physicians and those in leadership throughout the industry, the expansion of these boundaries results in a need for greater cognizance of morally ethical conduct to avoid conflicts of interest.

Physicians are expected to navigate many issues amid external and internal forces that influence critical decisions. The diverse environments in which physicians' practice must be understood within definable professional identities that transcend industry boundaries and traditional medical disciplines such that their professional role remains true to its traditional roots as healer/shaman from a sociological, ethical, and fiduciary perspective.

Hafferty and Castellani developed a model of a seven-cluster system of medical professionalism based on their work in complexity science.[27] In their study of the medical profession from a sociological perspective and through the lens of complexity science, they delineated the ways physicians seek to establish their own identity in their profession and society. They argued that these seven clusters of medical professionalism emerged in direct response to the historical forces of decentralization in which organized medicine has been situated for the past 30 years.

They viewed the historical forces of decentralization within the medical profession and within the complex system's distinction between organization and dynamics, such that the values, orientations, beliefs, specific skills, and ways of controlling the position within the larger bureaucratic structure are dynamically at play with one another in 10 key aspects of medical work that create competing clusters of professionalism: *autonomy, commercialism, social justice, social contract, altruism, professional dominance, technical competence, interpersonal competence, lifestyle ethic,* and *personal morality.*

Castellani and Hafferty use the complexity science agent-based processes such as *emergence, evolution, adaptation, feedback, autopoiesis, perturbation, self-organization,* and *operating far from equilibrium* to understand medical professionalism as a complex system. Applying network analysis, they identified the seven clusters as different ways of organizing medical work that uniquely combine and practice the 10 aspects of medical work in the complex system.

Each cluster is impacted by both internal and external forces that affect physicians as they grow into leaders or deeper in their clinical practice/research and the peer group they are engaged with over time. External forces such as managed care, consumerism, and health policy reform and internal forces such as health information technology, evidence-based medicine approaches to care processes, and challenges to authority and autonomy within complex organizations impact the development of professional identity.

Lifestyle Cluster. Physicians who identify with this cluster place strong values on nurturing family life and achieving a balance between their time at work and devotion to family, spiritual needs, and other interests. There is also a greater tendency to seek part-time or employed physician salaried positions.

As physician burnout rages on unabated, the emphasis on work-life balance around which some physicians define their professional identity is increasingly seen as a necessary and healthy approach to professionalism that contributes to resilience and ongoing professional satisfaction. With the advent of team-based care, telemedicine "gig" work, part-time opportunities, and job-sharing, alternative professional paths have expanded physicians' career opportunities that can incorporate a balanced approach to their life's work.

Entrepreneurial Cluster. Physicians in this cluster focus their efforts on improving the business model for healthcare service delivery. Innovations that lead to reductions in the cost of care and the waste of resources, improvement in quality, or expansion of services or products offered are highly important to these physicians.

While autonomy is key to this group, they recognize the transformation underway in healthcare, the need for greater collaboration, and shared authority in organizations. Although some perceive the decline in physician private practice as a decrease in their entrepreneurial role,[28] the ability to redesign healthcare delivery as part of a large clinical enterprise or in whole new delivery models enabled by digital technology will provide many opportunities for entrepreneurship within the medical profession in the coming years.

Unreflective Cluster. The focus of this cluster is on the day-to-day work that typifies episodic patient care. They may be disengaged from reform efforts, business model transformations, or research. The unreflective segment of the physician community tends to make no distinction between their personal and professional identity and may be particularly vulnerable during times of change.

Salaried employment models such as those offered by hospitals may be attractive to those who simply want to hunker down and see patients. However, Hafferty and Castellani's designation of such physicians as unreflective is more pejorative than necessary. Those who are focused on the technical aspects of their work, honing their skills and craft within the health system in which they practice, often lead in clinical excellence and outcomes. They may serve as the engineers of the profession, who continuously improve care delivery through their day-to-day focus on tactics.

Academic Cluster. The academic cluster attracts physicians who are the majority in the medical teaching ranks. Within this cluster, there are challenges to be reconciled. The presumed value placed by the academics on teaching is not reciprocated in financial compensation or tenure. The need to generate revenue from research competes with responsibilities of clinical practice within the academic environment, especially as the regulation in resident work hours and overall shortage in general surgery and general internal medicine squeeze the time to teach even further.

The industry has experienced a 4.2% reduction in the general surgeon workforce between 1981 and 2005.[29] This shortage continues, with the Association of American Medical Colleges predicting a shortage of 28,700 by 2033 for general surgeons[30] and a shortfall of up to 139,000 physicians across all specialties.[31]

The need to train more physicians will require a multipronged approach that includes redesigning the academic physician experience.

Activist Cluster. A group that is clearly focused on advancing the ideological needs of healthcare on local, national, and global scales is the activist cluster. The physician activist embraces the challenges of motivating peers and other stakeholders to support grassroots movements that can improve public health or the health of a particular population. With the onset of the pandemic, physicians have seen firsthand the impact of structural racism, inequality, and inadequate access to healthcare resources on the lives of their patients.

The AMA's Declaration of Professional Responsibility declares the members of the world community of physicians must commit to "advocate for social, economic, education, and political changes that ameliorate suffering and contribute to human wellbeing."

Since the murder of George Floyd by police officer Derek Chauvin and the subsequent intensification of Black Lives Matter advocacy, racism, not race itself, has been identified as a risk factor for disease. Many physicians have been motivated to become physician advocates to eliminate systemic racism and health inequities.

Advocacy is now understood not to be an elective pursuit for physicians but a professional obligation inculcated into the day-to-day clinical practice.[32]

Empirical Cluster. Physicians attracted to the empirical cluster are typically academic physicians who are research-oriented in contrast to those in academia who have a teaching focus. This group values the creation of new medical knowledge. The pressure to bring in research revenues to establish tenure may lead to a focus on safe, incremental approaches to science that lag in advancing evidence-based medicine practices, innovation of new medical technologies or therapies, or innovation in patient and population health models.

This group may be less concerned with idealistic movements in society but may still be marked by a strong sense of benevolence that must be balanced by their real need for grant-based revenues that often restrict radical approaches to scientific inquiry.

Nostalgic Cluster. Hafferty and Castellani consider the nostalgic group to be the most dominant of the seven clusters. This cluster tends to serve as a locus for those physicians operating at leadership levels across the industry in academic medical institutions, in medical societies, and in the production of medical publications.

As a collective, this group is focused on maintaining levels of autonomy and, while historically seen as fighting the commercialization of medicine, may have championed national movements such as the need for a transition away from the problematic fee-for-service model of reimbursement for care in exchange for a culture more driven by value-based purchasing initiatives, shared savings programs, and pay-for-performance incentive programs. Although they perceive that there may be problems or unintended consequences to work through in this transition,[33] as a whole, the aristocracy of medicine recognizes the need for change.

Although professional ethics should keep the interests of patients at the forefront of decision-making by physicians working in each of these seven clusters, the aspects of medical work that are most emphasized within an individual cluster are distinctive and therefore varying in leadership development implications.

Hafferty and Castellani identify key values in each of the seven clusters that define the professional behavior of physicians operating within the constructs of that cluster. The clusters can therefore be used to identify implications for leadership for physicians operating in each of the clusters (Figure 1).

For the nostalgic cluster, viewed as the ruling aristocracy of medicine, self-reflection regarding their idealized notions of the profession's past versus the

Professionalism Clusters	Value Guidepost	Leadership Implication
Academic	Teaching	Embraces the roles of training future physicians to prepare them for dealing with the continuous changes in healthcare.
Activist	Influencing	Engages in health reform campaigns and grassroots movements; recognizes that the need for the development of "influencing skills" is essential.
Empirical	Learning	Capitalizes on the opportunity to lead through the definition of what, how, and why resources are used for research.
Entrepreneurial	Innovating	Makes valuable reflections on the impact of disruptive innovation on the complexity of healthcare and ideas for improvement.
Lifestyle	Balancing	Must recognize the potential limitations for leadership development in lieu of their pursuit of work/life balance.
Nostalgic	Remembering	Viewed as the ruling aristocracy of medicine and self-reflective thought of the physician profession's past can be helpful in leadership.
Unreflective	Building	Engages in tactical day-to-day operations with a strong focus on health system improvement.

Figure 1.

dynamic changes of the contemporary professional will be useful. For the entrepreneurial physician, self-reflection on the impact of disruptive innovation on complex adaptive systems as it pertains to their ideal of improving care will be beneficial. Those in the academic cluster must parse their role in training future physicians with curriculum and culture change that prepares physicians for the changing healthcare system.

Physicians in the lifestyle cluster must reflect on the potential limitations to their personal leadership growth and development as they pursue the work/life balancing act that is increasingly complicated in contemporary American medicine. The empirical physician cluster offers the opportunity for physicians to lead by helping to define what, how, and why resources are used for research. The pertinence of effort becomes the guiding principle for leading in this group, such that research in system redesign and comparative effectiveness are emphasized.

The potential for strong engagement in health reform campaigns/public health grassroots movements for activist physicians is paramount, as long as physicians in this cluster understand the importance of bringing other physicians along in their efforts. Leadership development for activists involves skills in influencing others rather than simply fighting for pet causes.

Finally, the leadership for the so-called unreflective physician may involve engagement in those aspects of healthcare delivery that most influence their day-to-day work, such as care coordination, patient safety efforts, and workflow redesign.

These physicians should not be overlooked as leaders, for their willingness to work on system improvement at the micro-level will improve the likelihood of success in clinical integration efforts and population health management strategies.

These seven clusters have interesting implications for physician leadership development. The obligations physicians have not only to their patients, but in their wider professional roles with peers, clinical teams, students, and others in the industry necessitate self-reflection as to the pitfalls and potential opportunities implicit in the values embedded in each of the seven clusters.

Achieving health professionalism requires balancing one's personal needs with those of the community as it pertains to one's communal role.

PROFESSIONAL EXISTENTIALISM

The social and cultural changes in American post-industrial and information-centric society are transforming the role and status of physicians in radical ways. From a mid-20th-century position of high status, economic independence, and professional autonomy, physicians have moved into a world in which their traditional healing role is challenged by the complexity of contemporary healthcare organizations. David K. Zismer argues that "fully integrated health systems" must organize integrated (employed) physicians "within a system according to accepted principles and common expectations and policies" that are "accountable to a structure with a mission" in which physicians are "leaders and managers within the system design."

Zismer goes on to express that "Physicians' services must be optimized in pursuit of the goals of the health system overall." In such a system, physicians are "valued assets" of the system with "opportunities to play roles in care delivery design, organizational planning, and operations through an array of standing and ad hoc committees."[34]

In Zismer's model, physicians owe loyalty to "the system" and are "accountable to peers and the system for their professional behaviors." The physician's compensation is controlled by "a common employment agreement" at "market rates by clinical specialty" in which incentives "will align physicians with system goals and objectives."

Interestingly, Zismer notes that when physicians are sued for professional activities, "the organization is the first line of defense and support," revealing the disassociation of the individualistic approach to physician responsibility within the tort system to the ideals of the systems approach of integrated delivery systems

In the 2015 *JAMA* volume examining professionalism in the changing healthcare landscape, Jay Crosson, MD, presents an alternative construct for understanding physician professionalism in large group practices or in employed practices.

He notes that the Permanente Medical Group, the Mayo Clinic, and other historically successful large integrated physician groups are governed through physician self-regulation within a strong culture of group responsibility. These cultures and governance structures have produced high-quality patient services and satisfied patients. In general, these large group practice models are built on four key elements to physician self-regulation in the employment setting: clinical governance, management capabilities, clinical performance information transparency, and appropriateness of financial incentives.[35]

In contrast to Crosson's insights, Zismer's systems approach to understanding healthcare delivery does not recognize the existential core of the physician identity. Physicians' primary role is in their relationship to patients, not to an organizational system infrastructure. To be a physician is to be a healer, a social role as ancient as the shaman. Physicians have a social duty that is performed within the context of an existential relationship to an individual patient.

Prior to the Information Age, one of the key sources of strength in the relationship between physicians and their patients has been the asymmetries of information between the two. Physicians have been considered a trusted source of truth and knowledge girded in a social role focused on healing.

Despite the increased access to health information available to patients today, the identity of the physician as a sacred arbiter of sources of healing and comfort continues to supersede the obligations to an organization or system of care. The professional identity is an existential construct based on the duties of the physician to the patient, not to an organization. This covenant transcends time and place and may ultimately permit a renewal of physician authority as the ethical source of professional power, identity, and personal responsibility.

The moral obligations of professional self-regulation are built on the ethical responsibilities in the physician-patient relationship. Any broader delivery system obligations must be encompassed within the professional obligations to the patient, not *vice versa*.

The Cherokee word for health is "*tohi.*" *Tohi* is a communal concept in which living a balanced life contributes to the health of the entire community. The Cherokee word for living this balanced life is "*duyukdv.*" Within our Western context, living such a balanced life as a physician is intrinsic to professionalism and can provide an alternative model to traditional perceptions of physician work.

The health of the physician profession depends on balancing the needs of the individual physician with their fiduciary duties to their patients within the social and environmental conditions in which they practice their craft. The ability to prioritize the needs of others above one's own needs requires certain psychological strengths that are taxed by contemporary medical culture and training. Carrying the title of "physician" requires long-term choices that presume self-sacrifice and altruism, but currently convey less status and prestige than previously due to fundamental changes the profession is undergoing due to mostly external social and technological forces upon which there is little professional control.

Hospitals, health plans, and public sector payers all exert legal, regulatory, contractual, and accreditation requirements for the oversight of clinical care. A physician's inability to discern the implicit paradox of the cultural expectation of their social role may contribute to the inability to take on the leadership roles required to be effective in the transformation of the healthcare system to one that is more functional, equitable, and sustainable. Communal health depends on achieving professional wellbeing. Physicians may require a new sense of existential wellbeing in order to take on the leadership roles necessary to serve our patients and communities.

James Madera, MD, links professionalism directly to the IOM's Triple Aim of better health, better healthcare, and lower cost. He notes that there exists a "set of moral values that guide as well as constrain the physician's behavior including altruism, integrity, caring, and community focus" that must adapt to the rapidly changing healthcare system" while maintaining self-regulation.

He sees medical professionalism built on self-regulation built on three fundamental elements: (1) agreed-upon standards by which individuals may enter the profession and by which they then practice, (2) responsibility for teaching these professionals how to exercise those standards on a day-to-day basis, and (3) enforcing those standards and deciding when and how those who violated them will be disciplined.

By embracing changes that reflect new priorities and attitudes toward healthcare delivery and the health of the population, professionalism expands beyond a physicians' individual behavior and embraces the goals and vision embedded in the Triple Aim.[36]

PROFESSIONALISM IN INDUSTRY RELATIONS

Now that the majority of physicians work in paid positions of regular employment of large medical centers, healthcare corporations, and payer-owned companies, the ongoing professional obligation either directly or indirectly to patients is at risk of being obscured by other social contracts built on traditional business models rather than a traditional doctor-patient relationship.

The aim of each physician should continue to be the care for and protection of the interests and wellbeing of patients to the best of that physician's abilities, irrespective of business obligations. Whether organized as a for-profit or not-for-profit business, all health-related businesses need to remain economically sustainable, and healthcare company leaders have fiduciary responsibilities to maintain their financial bottom line.

There is something different about medicine, however. While healthcare business may focus on shareholders and profit because that is how companies are thought to contribute most to overall social welfare, physicians' responsibilities originate not from broader social welfare but from a commitment to the individual patient.[37] Fiduciary duty is an obligation to act in the best interest of another person or party. The fiduciary is entrusted with the care of another person and must ensure that the person's interests take precedence over the fiduciary's own interests.

Fiduciary duty for physicians is embedded in their relationship to patients. In business, executives have a fiduciary duty to the shareholders of the corporation. Can physicians maintain two fiduciary duties simultaneously, to both patients and a business interest? Broader medical professionalism that expands fiduciary duty to symbiotically design and organize around efficiency, profit, advancing medical science, and patient care can be built on cultures and processes that acknowledge the tensions between medical and business approaches while maintaining a trustee relationship to in all fiduciary obligations.

Physicians must ensure that they continue to lead continuous process improvement to improve quality and enhance innovation as new discoveries and healthcare delivery systems evolve. Physician relations with industry are important to advancing science and the development of new services and interventions for patient care. However, physician leaders must monitor relations for themselves, their organizations, and the broader physician community to ensure that four objectives are met:

1. Ensuring ethical conduct.
2. Prohibiting fraud.
3. Properly handing remuneration.
4. Avoiding conflicts of interest.

Regardless of whether it is a small physician group practice, integrated health system, radiology center, clinically integrated network, or a public health program, each organization places physicians squarely in contact with other stakeholders across the industry. Within the broader healthcare ecosystem, patterns of relationships are established, and some fuel sustainability of programs and organizations while others may lead to the self-organization of new entities.

In 1994, Dr. David Blumenthal noted three key elements to strengthen professionalism: *altruism, self-improvement,* and *peer review.*[38] When focused on with the proper resources and effort, each of these elements can help ensure the accomplishment of the four objectives in their impact on relations with industry.

Physicians have interactions with industry in several different sectors, including biotechnology, health policy development, health information technology, managed care, and medical device manufacturers. The vendors and organizations that provide services and products across these sectors need physicians in development, validation, and testing stages to advance and introduce new interventions across markets. Physician executives and practicing physicians must manage all of these relations with the utmost scrutiny. The Stark Law provides physicians with rules that govern self-referral patterns and relationships, while the Anti-kickback Statute put in place guardrails to deter the occurrence of fraud and abuse that impacts patients and federal health programs negatively.

As physician leaders address emergent health reforms, these statutory frameworks provide guidance that reinforces the importance of professionalism in physician-to-industry relations. Physicians' role on advisory boards and recruitment of patients for new pharmaceutical/biotechnology trials is important to the advancement of medical innovation. Whether physicians play a role in leadership and governance, the importance of meeting the four objectives is part of professional responsibility.

Ensuring Ethical Conduct. Maintaining and enforcing ethical conduct in industry and vendor relations is critical to physician leaders' efforts to successfully improve the quality of care their organizations deliver. The ethical conduct of physician activities in the field of research is especially critical in the administration of human subject involvement. Physicians drive much of this activity both in the academic medical sector and in the private sector through physician practice recruitment of human subjects.

The huge financial risks and rewards at stake in medical research make physicians' duty to ensure optimal patient safety all the more critical. The "avoidance of research malfeasance and unethical treatment of human subjects" is an absolute standard for professional behavior.[39]

There is tremendous pressure for revenue and income generation, given the decrements that physicians have experienced over the past decade with the transition away from the fee-for-service reimbursement model in moving toward pay-for-performance and value-based purchasing models for compensation. However, in the quest to achieve optimal financial performance for healthcare organizations, physician leaders make it a priority in tactical planning to enforce policies that govern the ethical conduct in industry relations and research activities.

Prohibiting Fraud. Fraudulent activities in patient care operations are an unfortunate but real occurrence. Physicians' professionalism is compromised when they submit to any pressures that result in engagement in fraud. For the physician leader, it is essential to have appropriate organizational and financial controls in place to monitor for any fraudulent activities. Public trust is compromised and professional authority is further tarnished with the occurrence of even a single event.

Remuneration for Physicians. Federal regulations often focus on the necessity of compensating physicians at "fair market value," which is, unfortunately, narrowly defined by the current value of physicians' services in terms of relative value unit (RVU)-based evaluation and management and current procedural terminology (CPT) coding. This approach does not take into account the arbitrary and political nature of valuation based on productivity-based work units and contributes to the devaluation of the larger role of physicians in healthcare and diminishes the ability of physicians to be valued for their managerial and leadership functions.

With the prolonged years of training, diminished professional status, and employment models based on obsolete accounting methodologies, physicians are paradoxically in short supply but underpaid relative to market demand, leading to shortages in physician supply in primary care, general surgery, and other specialties in which "the net present value of becoming a physician may become negative."[40] In such an environment, there is considerable risk in unethical arrangements for physician remuneration from research and other industry activities that must be acknowledged and ethically challenged.

In the sector of research activities, compensation for the recruitment of patients for participation in clinical trials is governed by industry guidance. Along these lines, the AMA offers guidance to physicians engaging in research in both the private and academic sector of the industry:

> Any remuneration received by the researcher from the company whose product is being studied must be commensurate with the efforts of the researcher on behalf of the company.[41]

Remuneration is an issue that can affect brand loyalty[42] of some surgeons and physicians in the selection and usage of therapeutics and devices, so there is an inherent need to monitor for conflicts of interest along with ensuring that the level of remuneration is commensurate with the level of physician effort.

In addition to patient recruitment, conducting clinical trials as investigators and preparing reports on research findings are also activities in which physicians have compensation arrangements with industry.

Physicians in both private practice and academic medicine face a variety of challenges in managing compensation. Physician leaders have a need to understand those challenges to help navigate the changes with health reforms at federal and state levels that impact remuneration in patient care, research, and other revenue-generating activities that physicians may participate in on a regular basis.

Conflicts of Interest. Key to the successful management of every physician's relations with industry stakeholders is avoiding any conflicts of interest. Physicians are considered fiduciaries in their relationship with their patients and the healthcare organizations for which they provide services. In 2009, the IOM defined a conflict of interest as:

> . . . a set of circumstances that creates a risk that professional judgment or actions regarding a primary interest will be unduly influenced by a secondary interest.[43]

The IOM emphasizes that the primary interests may be construed as patient care, medical education, and research integrity, while secondary interests are primarily determined to be financial interests. The secondary interest must not create any unnecessary or unethical influence on professional/clinical decisions regarding patient care or for the physician's organization that provides care delivery services.

A number of critical elements must be maintained throughout each relationship with industry vendors to ensure proper management and avoidance of conflicts of interest, including:

- Balancing loyalties by placing the patient first in professional and clinical decision making that affects their wellbeing.
- Maintaining objectivity and impartiality to avoid any unethical influence.
- Ensuring that trust is not compromised.
- Ensuring that personal gains are not sought.[44]

Physician leaders must ensure that effective controls are in place within their organizations to monitor conflicts of interest to ensure that public/patient trust is maintained. However, the complete avoidance of conflicts of interest is not desirable. Often those with the most expertise inherently have greater conflicts of interest.

For example, an advisory board of a biomedical company will be stronger with medical scientists who have experience in the biotech industry than one made up of random clinicians. The work of that advisory board should be remunerated. Conflicts of interest cannot be completed avoided. Instead, they should be acknowledged transparently and sometimes openly considered as part of the governance and decision-making processes of all healthcare businesses.

For physicians, acknowledging patient fiduciary obligations and business ones can strengthen rather than weaken professional contributions. By expanding fiduciary duties to not only include a commitment to the individual patient but also a commitment to overall social welfare and acknowledging inherent conflicts of interest in business and expanded roles, physicians can lead with distinctive and special responsibility.

REDEMPTION

Renewing professionalism across the physician community will require involvement from all medical disciplines. In doing so, professional identities will be reshaped while physician leaders manage and mitigate risks and promote their organizations' missions.

The path from hero to leader embraces the concept of a new professionalism. This new professionalism is one that drives physicians toward a community focus needed in managing the health of a population and will develop physician leaders who understand the need to transition from the individualistic and heroic model of care and embrace the path of caring for the population and community as a whole.

The overarching principle that links the seven professional clusters is a consensus that an ongoing fiduciary duty drives the need for right behavior as healers and servants necessary for physicians to embody as they lead and manage the 21st-century healthcare system.

REFERENCES

1. Freidson E. *Professionalism: The Third Logic*, Chicago, IL: The University of Chicago Press; 2007, p. 213.
2. Freidson, p. 17.
3. Mitchell SW. *Doctor and Patient*. Philadelphia, PA: J.P. Lippincott Company. 1988. Reprinted special edition, Classics of Medicine Library. Bethesda, MD: Gryphon Editions;1994, p. 43.
4. Mitchell, pp. 43-48.
5. Mitchell, p. 53.
6. Jonsen AR, Mark Siegler M, Winslade WJ. *Clinical Ethics: A Practical Approach to Ethical Decisions in Clinical Medicine*, 2nd Ed. New York, NY: Macmillan Publishing; 1986, p. 12.
7. Beauchamp TL, Childress JF. *Principles of Biomedical Ethics*, 4th ed. New York, NY: Oxford University Press; 1994, pp. 395-461.
8. Beauchamp, p. 502.
9. Beauchamp, p. 48.
10. Beauchamp, pp. 494-5.
11. Freidson, pp. 116-17.
12. Freidson, p. 149.
13. Freidson, p. 149.
14. Freidson, p. 117.

15. Freidson, p. 121.

16. Freidson, p. 116.

17. Freidson, p. 139.

18. Beauchamp, p. 464.

19. American Medical Association. Declaration of Professional Responsibility. Medicine's Social Contract With Humanity. Adopted by House of Delegates of the American Medical Association on December 4, 2001.

20. Baron RJ. Professional Self-regulation in a Changing World: Old Problems Need New Approaches. *JAMA*.2015;313(18):1807-8. doi:10.1001/jama.2015.4060.

21. Emanuel EJ. Enhancing Professionalism Through Management. *JAMA*. 2015:313(18): 1799-1800.doi.10.1001/jama.2015.4336.

22. Baron, p. 1807.

23. Emanuel, p. 1799.

24. Abbott A. *The System of Professions: An Essay on the Division of Expert Labor.* Chicago, IL: University of Chicago Press; 1988, p. 188.

25. Leicht KT, Fennell ML. Change in the Organizational Context of Managerial and Professional Work. In: *Professional Work: A Sociological Approach.* Oxford, UK: Blackwell Publishers; 2001, pp. 96-132.

26. Leicht, p. 174.

27. Hafferty FW, Castellani B. The Increasing Complexities of Professionalism. *Academic Medicine.* 2010;85(2):288-301.

28. Fuchs VR. The Transformation of US Physicians. JAMA. 2015;(18):1821-22. doi:10.1001/jama.2015.2915.

29. Kavic M. Professionalism, Passion, and Surgical Education *JSLS*. 2010 Jul-Sep;14(3):321-4.

30. Welsh DJ, et.al. 2019 ACS Governors Survey: Surgeons Wanted: Workforce Challenges in Health Care. Bulletin of the American College of Surgeons. July 21, 2020. bulletin.facs.org.

31. Association of American Medical Colleges. The Complexities of Physician Supply and Demand: Projections from 2018 to 2033.. Association of American Medical Colleges. June 2020. aamc.org.

32. Ojo A, Sandoval RS, Soled D, Stewart A. No Longer an Elective Pursuit: The Importance of Physician Advocacy in Everyday Medicine. Health Affairs Blog, August 19, 2020. 10.1377/hblog2020817.667867.

33. Mehrotra A, Sorbero ME, Damberg CL Using the Lessons of Behavioral Economics to design More Effective Pay-for-Performance Programs. *Am J Manag Care.* 2010 Jul;16(7):497-503.

34. Zismer DK. The Psychology of Organizational Structure in Integrated Health Systems. *Physician Exec.* 2011 May-June;37(3):36-43.

35. Crosson FJ. Physician Professionalism in Employed Practice. *JAMA*. 2015;313(18):1817-18. doi:10.1001/jama.2015.3742.

36. Madera JL, Burkhardt. Professionalism, Self-regulation, and Motivation: How Did Health Care Get This So Wrong? *JAMA*. 2015;313(18):1793-94. Doi:10.1001/jama.2015.4045.

37. Margolis JD. Professionalism, Fiduciary Duty, and Health-Related Business Leadership. *JAMA*. 2015(18):1819-20. Doi:10.1001/jama.2015.4398.
38. Blumenthal D. The Vital Role of Professionalism in Health Care Reform. *Health Aff (Millwood)*. 1994 Spring;13(1):252-6.
39. Fisher JA. Practicing Research Ethics: Private-sector Physicians & Pharmaceutical Clinical Trials *Soc Sci Med*. 2008;66(12):2495–05.
40. Papadimos TJ, Hartner RL, Marco AP. Cyclical vs. Structural Economic Weakness; The Effects on Physician Mobility and Recruiting. *Physician Exec*. 2011 May-June;37(3):18-22.
41. American Medical Association Code of Medical Ethics. Opinion 8.031—Conflicts of Interest: Biomedical Research. physician-resources/medical-ethics/code-medical-ethics/opinion8031.page? #.
42. Robinson JC. Applying Value-based Insurance Design to High-cost Health Services. *Health Aff (Millwood)*. 2010;29(11):2009-16.
43. Institute of Medicine. Committee on Conflict of Interest in Medical Research, Education, and Practice. *Conflict of Interest In Medical Research, Education, and Practice*. Washington, DC: National Academies Press (US); 2009, p. 46.
44. Institute of Medicine, pp. 6-7.

CHAPTER 7: PROFESSIONALISM IS REDEMPTION

Leadership Implications and Health Policy Considerations

Leadership Implications:

1. Establish a system of controls that signal when incidents occur that negatively impact meeting the four objectives in industry relations.
2. Reflect upon which professional clusters are pertinent in your own career.

Health Policy Considerations:

1. Understand leadership opportunities for physicians aligned within various clusters (as part of the professional topology of the physician community) and how to impact the development of policy options for ethical conduct and avoiding conflicts of interest.
2. In development of policies governing conflicts of interest over physician relations with industry, ensure that each is evaluated for proportionality, transparency, accountability, and fairness.

Physician Generation Next

"Whatever you can do, or dream you can, begin it. Boldness has genius, power, and magic in it."[1]

Johann Wolfgang von Goethe

Physicians who are focused on improving the U.S. healthcare system are overcoming challenges and improving outcomes through efforts to redesign how care is accessed, paid for, and provided. The expectations for the next generation of healthcare leaders are high and will require a great deal of effort to transition the industry to a new level of operational excellence.

From coast to coast, great programs and organizations led by physicians working hand in hand with multidisciplinary teams are improving the quality of direct patient care services and the overall administration of health systems and physician practices. These improvement goals have become established in the overarching framework of the "Triple Aim":[2]

1. Better care for individuals.
2. Better health for populations.
3. Lower growth in expenditures.

For years, the Triple Aim has served as the lodestone for much of the improvement initiatives across the U.S. healthcare system in the public and private sector. Yet, much remains unaccomplished in broadly achieving these aspirations. With this in mind, breaking through the impasses constraining the healthcare delivery system will require far-reaching changes in how healthcare is provided and how physicians lead.

The focus of the preceding chapters has been the implications of this cultural transformation to better prepare physicians for the necessary leadership journey. This book develops three overarching themes.

First is the ongoing need for *innovation* in contemporary medicine, in both professional roles and system design. Transformed physician leadership will be critical to the successful conceptualization and implementation of new interventions, models, and systems that improve the quality of care.

Second, understanding historic difficulties in improving the efficiency and effectiveness of health services is framed within the language of *complexity theory*. No unique villain has led to our current system's inadequacies. Rather, complex adaptive systems evolve. Without understanding how complex adaptive systems operate, leaders will fail to recognize and mitigate unintended outcomes in their attempts to address organizational problems.

The science of predictive modeling in advanced systems can improve reliability and thus improve care in complex systems such as integrated delivery systems, academic medical centers, multispecialty medical groups, or medical homes. More importantly, the ongoing fiduciary responsibilities embedded in a physician's professional role can serve as an immutable principle that supersedes particular circumstances. The redemptive quality of professionalism has the capability to inculcate evolution rather than devolution in the complex adaptive systems in which healthcare is delivered.

The third theme is the evolving *path to leadership* for physicians in the rapidly changing healthcare system. Physician leaders may develop their skills by undergoing a paradigmatic shift in perspective, from playing an isolating heroic role that does not function well in complex adaptive systems to becoming a professional whose duties and actions are integrated in a health-centric manner in the community they serve.

This new professionalism emphasizes the ongoing relationship between the health of individual patients, the health of the physician, and the health of the community in which both reside. The importance of collaboration across the entire healthcare ecosystem and the broader community in which it resides is essential, and physicians who engage and lead efforts that positively impact the systems and underlying processes will do so with their clinical, technical, business, and strategic skills.

INNOVATION TODAY

The publication of *To Err Is Human* in 1999 heralded a growing dissatisfaction with the status quo in the healthcare industry by shattering the illusion that the U.S. healthcare industry was of high quality second to none. Subsequently, we have seen a renaissance of sorts in the industry with a reengineering of delivery system models and quality management processes coupled with discoveries and advancements of biomedical technology.

Remote health monitoring systems, point-of-service clinical decision support tools, artificial intelligence-designed diagnostic technologies, and new nanotechnologies that improve health technology instrumentation are driving solutions less dependent on high-cost, facility-based healthcare delivery.

Over the last 20 years, there has been increasing recognition that an unfettered fee-for-service payment system is a major culprit in the high-cost, inadequate quality nature of the delivery system. The Affordable Care Act (2009), MACRA (2015), and 21st Century Cures Act (2016) have strengthened the industry focus on value delivered across the spectrum of patient care services, bringing to the market new innovations in care delivery, biotechnology, and information science.

Innovation in patient care delivery models and comparative effectiveness research is being driven by the expectation that there will be a significant return on investment for those who bring more efficiency to the market.

For every challenge in healthcare today, there are opportunities to uncover breakthroughs that advance the quality of care delivered. But as Clayton Christensen pointed out, innovation is intrinsically disruptive.[3]

The complexity of the healthcare delivery system creates an environment in which innovative solutions to problems do not always easily fit into the system. The capital outlay for financing technology, third-party payers, and the highly regulated environment are not necessarily conducive to rapid transfer to evidence-based, point-of-care solutions.

Disruptive innovations arrive in the healthcare mainstream market clumsily, although the penetration of retail medical clinics, telemedicine, electronic health records, and pharmacogenomics do indicate adoption of innovations in the healthcare market is accelerating. Incremental improvement has been more the rule in delivery system transformation due to the inherent conservatism of the third-party payer system. However, the Affordable Care Act created enough disruption in the insurance industry to accelerate the pace of change.

In 2006, the Institute of Medicine organized the Roundtable on Evidence-based Medicine (now known as the Roundtable on Value & Science-Driven Health Care), which conducted workshops focused on issues pertinent to improvement in the science of medical practice. In 2010, the roundtable released *Redesigning the Clinical Effectiveness Research Paradigm: Innovation and Practice-Based Approaches: Workshop Summary*, which summarized the workshop presentations.[4]

REDESIGNING THE CLINICAL EFFECTIVENESS RESEARCH PARADIGM
• Address limitations in applicability of research results.
• Define strategic use of the clinical experimental model.
• Encourage innovation in clinical effectiveness research.
• Promote effectiveness research as a routine part of practice.
• Improve access/use of clinical data acknowledge resource.
• Forster transformational research potential of information technology.
• Engage patients as full partners in the learning culture.

Figure 1.

From the presentations, a number of themes emerged on how the science of medical practice should be redesigned to be more clinically effective.[5] Many of the themes articulated at the workshop (Figure 1) have subsequently been embedded in the health reform legislation.

Key to the redesign efforts for physicians in practice and in healthcare services administration is the opportunity to close the gap between science and bedside care, leading to an improved quality of life for many patients.

As the efforts of this roundtable and other groups fed into the national health and science policy development framework, ARRA put in place the language to launch a new long-term comparative effectiveness research program on a national scale. Its purpose is to validate the comparability of existing and new medications, interventions, and tools for use by physicians and patients. The Patient Centered Outcomes Research Institute (PCORI) was established to lead research from this new perspective. ARRA appropriated $1.1 billion for PCORI.

PCORI's focus has been to compare outcomes to determine the effectiveness, including risk and benefits, of two or more approaches to healthcare. Comparative clinical effectiveness research examines strategies for prevention, screening diagnosis, treatment, or management of clinical conditions, methods to improve the delivery of care, interventions to reduce or eliminate disparities in heat, and health communication techniques.

The focus of the grants are conditions that affect large numbers of people across a range of populations; conditions that place a heavy burden on individuals, families, specific populations, and society; and rare diseases.

Particular attention focuses on racial and ethnic minorities, older adults, low-income people, residents of rural areas, women, children, individuals with disabilities, people with multiple chronic diseases, patients with low health literacy/numeracy or limited English proficiency, LGBT persons, and veterans and members of the armed forces.[6]

Since it began operations in 2012, PCORI has funded hundreds of studies that compare healthcare options to learn which works best, given patients' circumstances and preferences.

Initially controversial, PCORI was refunded in 2020 with broad bipartisan support for an additional 10 years at $150 million annually. Its reauthorization changed the language of PCORI's statute with explicit mentions about its responsibility for research to consider the economic burden of interventions on patients, including out-of-pocket costs.[7]

Despite the ongoing work of PCORI, clinically effective, cost-efficient innovation diffuses slowly in the current delivery system. Fuchs and Milstein argue that the reason for this slow adoption of innovation is multifactorial and fueled by "perceptions and behaviors of major participants in health care."[8] They note that hospital administrators have faced financial challenges due to the enormous capital acquisition costs for technology at a time in which the industry is transitioning to outpatient service delivery models. Likewise, they note that physicians are challenged by fears that changes brought on by innovation will have adverse impacts on their practices, compensation, and autonomy.

The 2015 MACRA legislation created the Physician-focused Technical Advisory Committee (PTAC) in part to improve how the Medicare program pays physicians for the care they provide to Medicare beneficiaries (Figure 2). PTAC encourages the development of alternative payment models, referred to as physician-focused payment models, by making comments and recommendations to the Secretary of the Department of Health and Human Services on proposals submitted to PTAC by individuals and stakeholder entities. PTAC allows input into Medicare payment policy directly from physicians and other stakeholders in the field.[9]

Since its inception, PTAC has received more than 40 proposals and provided input directly to the Secretary on 28 of them at the time of this writing (Figure 3). The breadth of innovation in the proposals coming directly from practicing providers indicates the capacity for design thinking the provider community is capable of when coupled with appropriate methods of support.

- PTAC was created to contribute to a national priority to improve the efficiency and effectiveness of the U.S. health care delivery system. We believe that proposed solutions from frontline stakeholders in our delivery system can substantially enhance quality, improve affordability and influence policy development and system transformation.
- PTAC providers a forum where those in the field may directly convey both their ideas and their concerns on how to deliver high-value care for Medicare beneficiaries and others seeking health care services in our nation. PTAC is committed to ensuring our stakeholders have access to independent, expert input and that their perspectives and innovations reach the Secretary of Health and Human Services.
- PTAC will continue to submit comments and recommendations regarding physician-focused payment models submitted by stakeholders to the Secretary, as required by statute. In addition, we will expand our communications with the Centers for Medicare & Medicaid Services (CMS) and stakeholders to identify opportunities to further inform and prioritize the work CMS, including the Center for Medicare & Medicaid Innovation (CMMI), and other policymakers are undertaking to modernize healthcare.

Figure 2. PTAC Vision Statement

- The "Medical Neighborhood" Advanced Alternative Payment Model
- Patient-Centered Oncology Payment Model (CPOP)
- Eye Care Emergency Department Avoidance (EyEDA)
- Patient-Centered Asthma Care Payment
- ACCESS Telemedicine: An Alternative Healthcare Delivery Model for Rural Cerebral Emergencies
- CAPABLE Provider Focused Payment Model
- CMS Support of Wound Care in Private Outpatient Therapy Clinics: Measuring the Effectiveness of Physical or Occupational Therapy Intervention as the Primary Means of Managing Wounds in Medicare Recipients

Figure 3. Proposals to PTAC Evaluated and Reported to the Secretary:

(continues next page)

- Bundled Payment for All-Inclusive Outpatient Wound Care Services in Non-Hospital Based Setting
- Making Accountable Sustainable Oncology Networks (MASON)
- Acute Unscheduled Care Model (AUCM): Enhancing Appropriate Admissions
- Comprehensive Care Physician Payment Model
- An Innovative Model for Primary Care Office Payment
- Alternative Payment Model for Improved Quality and Cost in Providing Home Hemodialysis to Geriatric Patients Residing in Skilled Nursing Facilities
- Intensive Care Management in Skilled Nursing Facility Alternative Payment Model (ICM SNF APM)
- Home Hospitalization: An Alternative Payment Model for Delivering Acute Care in the Home
- Patient and Caregiver Support for Serious Illness
- Advanced Care Model (ACM) Service Delivery and Advanced Alternative Payment Model
- Incident ESRD Clinical Episode Payment Model
- Multi-provider, bundled episode-of-care payment model for treatment of chronic hepatitis C virus (HCV) using care coordination by employed physicians in hospital outpatient clinics
- Medicare 3-Year Value-Based Payment Plan (Medicare 3VPBP)
- Annual Wellness Visit Billing at Rural Health Clinics
- Advanced Primary Care: A Foundational Alternative Payment Model (APC/APM)
- LUGPA APM for Initial Therapy of Newly Diagnosed Patients with Organ-Confined Prostate Cancer
- Oncology Bundled Payment Program Using CAN-Guided Care
- "HaH Plus" (Hospital at Home Plus) Provider-Focused Payment Model
- Project Sonar
- The COPD and Asthma Monitoring Project
- The ACS-Brandeis Advanced APM

Figure 3. *(continued)* **Proposals to PTAC Evaluated and Reported to the Secretary:**

The Medicare and Medicaid Center for Innovation (Innovation Center) was established by the Patient Protection and Affordable Care Act in order to test innovative payment and delivery system models that show promise for maintaining or improving the quality of care in Medicare, Medicaid, and the Children's Health Insurance Program (CHIP), while slowing the rate of growth in program costs.

The Innovation Center is chartered to test, evaluate, and diffuse new programs with the promise of improving care coordination, payment and reimbursement models, population health management models, and overall communication and quality involved in patient care. The center is statutorily required to prioritize 20 models specified in the law, including medical homes, all-payer payment reform, and arrangements that transition from fee-for-service reimbursement to global fees and salary-based payment.

If a CMMI pilot model is considered successful, the Secretary of Health and Human Services may expand its duration and scope. As pilot programs are funded, those that prove successful will have the opportunity to be further explored and tested on a broader basis regionally and nationally. Projects will disperse across three areas identified by the Innovation Center in 2011:[10]

1. Patient Care Models
2. Seamless Coordination Models
3. Community and Population Health Models

In the past 10 years, CMMI has launched 54 payment and service delivery models designed to transform the American healthcare system from one that pays for volume to one that pays for value. Currently, 40% of Medicare fee-for-service payments, 30% of commercial payments, and 25% of Medicaid payments are being made through some form of value-based arrangement.[11]

The success of CMMI is controversial. Gross savings that are calculated with the use of the model benchmarks are on average 235% higher than gross savings calculated in independent evaluation with the use of a retrospective control group.[12]

In 2021, Accountable Care Organizations have grown to 477 Medicare ACOs and hundreds more affiliated with private payers. Medicare ACOs alone serve 10.7 million beneficiaries and have saved Medicare $8.5 billion in gross savings and $2.5 billion in net savings.[13]

THE ONGOING PHYSICIAN LEADERSHIP JOURNEY

The healthcare delivery system is complex, changing rapidly, and far from physician-centric or physician-friendly in its current iteration. To improve the healthcare delivery system, it must be understood as a complex adaptive system in which physician leadership is obligatory for its success. This leadership draws on the traditional sacred power in the healer role, the ethical bond to the patient underlying the physician's place in the community at large.

The path to leadership is a developmental one and should be built on a model of professional behavior for physicians where one lives one's life with truth and dignity. Professional integrity for physicians must be based on a role in the community that provides health and balance. From shaman to hero to contemporary leader, powerful healers must address the health of the society in which they live.

Intrinsic Motivation. One does not happen to become a physician. An individual must have the desire or ability to take on the role. It is a competitive process that requires perseverance, delayed gratification, analytic intelligence, self-abnegation, but also self-confidence. At its best, it is a servant leader role.

The Education. The education of a physician requires four years of college, four years of medical school, then 3–10 years of post-graduate training in order to develop the clinical skills necessary for the competent practice of medicine. Medical education henceforth must also integrate those skills necessary for physician leadership beyond diagnostic, evaluation, and treatment skills currently emphasized. Effective communication, strategy and tactics, management, team-building skills, systems theory, and process improvement skills are equally important.

The Experience. Medicine is a practice. It is a daily application of one's skills within the context of one's social identity and obligation to serve the needs of patients. It is a one-on-one experience. In each encounter with each patient, there is a unique duty. The broadening of a physician's duty to larger social obligations inherent in leadership requires the application of wisdom learned from these individual encounters to guide one's actions in the wider context.

Convergence. Convergence is a point in the journey where physicians are able to amalgamate their erudition acquired from both education and experience. At this stage, the benefits of experience from the clinical and technical perspective start to benefit physicians in the shaping of their careers as leaders, so long as they are cognizant of their obligation to the community as a whole.

A New Professionalism. Existential professionalism balances one's personal needs with the necessary obligation to the patient and to the community as a whole. Maslow's "self-actualization" as a developmental stage becomes possible only when one's basic needs are first fulfilled.

Within the context of the professional role, a physician can be self-actualized in leadership, which focuses not simply on the one-to-one relationship to an individual patient, but within one's role and responsibility to society as a whole. This transformation involves the existential realization of one's social role outside the constraints of the doctor-patient individual obligations.

Leadership involves expanding these duties to the community. In a world in which health care is improved through systems of care, teams of professionals, and collaborative care over a continuum, it will be critical to physician identity.

LET'S GET READY

The role of the healer is a powerful role. It is also the role of a servant. In the complex environment of contemporary healthcare, physicians find themselves at a critical juncture in history that beacons a call for leadership across the profession.

Since the medical community responds to emergencies both locally and internationally without hesitation, the entire profession must respond to the urgency of the healthcare system reform with as much passion as that displayed on the front lines of the COVID epidemic.

The simultaneous obligation to individual patients and to the community as a whole is a reorientation from the traditional clinical role and requires new skills, but the same perseverance and ethical commitment to healing is pertinent. Healthy communities require healthy leaders.

We need to be ready. Retail clinics, telemedicine, remote patient monitoring, alternative payment models, team-based care, artificial intelligence, whole-genome sequencing based life plans, precision medicine, virtual-reality based therapy, advances in longevity science, advanced robotics, care anywhere anytime, pandemics, climate change, social justice, integrated community care models, radiological images with images as precise as tissue under the microscope, microbiome diagnostics and therapeutics, predictive modeling as prevention medicine are already here, just not distributed evenly. We must lead.

REFERENCES

1. Goethe J. *Goethe's Faust*. New York: Anchor Publishing; 1962.

2. Center for Medicare & Medicaid Services. CMS-1345-P, Medicare Program; Medicare Shared Savings Program: Accountable Care Organizations. Proposed Rule. I(A). Introduction and Overview of Value-Based Purchasing. March 31, 2011.

3. Christensen CM, Raynor ME. The Disruptive Innovation Model. In: *The Innovator's Solution: Creating and Sustaining Successful Growth*. Boston, MA: Harvard Business School Publishing Corporation; 2003, pp. 32-35.

4. Institute of Medicine, Roundtable on Value & Science-Driven Health Care. Summary. In: *Redesigning the Clinical Effectiveness Research Paradigm. Innovation and Practice-Based Approaches Workshop Summary*. Washington, DC: National Academies Press; 2010, p. 11.

5. Institute of Medicine, p. 11.

6. Patient-Centered Outcomes Research Institute. Pcori.org.

7. Castellucci M. 10 Years After Inception, Industry Backs The Federal Research Institute. Modern Healthcare. March 14, 2020. modernhealthcare.com.

8. Fuchs VR, Milstein A. The $640 Billion Question—Why Does Cost-effective Care Diffuse So Slowly? *N Engl J Med*. 2011;364(21):1985-7.

9. Office of the Assistant Secretary for Planning and Evaluation, U.S. Department of Health and Human Services. aspe.hhs.gov

10. Center for Medicare & Medicaid Services. Center for Medicare and Medicaid Innovation's Seamless and Coordinated Care Models. http://innovations.cms.gov/areas-of-focus/seamless-and-coordinated-care-models.

11. Health Care Payment Learning & Action Network. APM Measurement: Progress of Alternative Payment Models: 2019 Methodology and Results Report. HCPLAN. 2019. http://hcp-lan.org/workproducts/apm-methodology-2019.pdf.

12. Smith B. CMS Innovation Center at 10 Years—Progress and Lessons Learned. *N Engl J Med*. 2021;384:759-64 dOI: 10.1056/NEJMsb2031138.

13. National Association of ACOs. naacos.com.

CHAPTER 8: PHYSICIAN GENERATION NEXT
Leadership Implications and Health Policy Considerations

Leadership Implications:

1. Examine your intrinsic motivations in designing your personal leadership journey.
2. Consider what impact on healthcare quality and outcomes you can make within your current professional role.

Health Policy Considerations:

1. Consider how inadequate preparedness for the global pandemic determined a trajectory leading to worldwide illness, death, and economic turmoil and related this to future leadership and policy responsibilities for the medical profession.
2. Analyze the implications of the accelerating pace of technological and culture change within th context of medical professionalism and the traditional role of healer.

PART III:

Leadership Profiles in Action

CHAPTER 9

Real Physicians, Real Leaders

This book is a revision of an effort I made 12 years ago to think through the implications of the rapid changes in the healthcare delivery system landscape and how I foresaw it impacting the medical profession. I began by reflecting on the profession's developmental history and moved to thinking about the impact of technology, policy, and cultural changes. I explored some of the academic frameworks on leadership and professionalism in the sociology literature and applied it in my analysis.

I also profiled three physicians I had had the privilege of knowing and whom I admired for their leadership and professionalism. Eugenie Komives, MD, Eliot Williams, MD, and Alan Kaplan, MD, illustrate the leadership frameworks of situational leadership, servant leadership, and transformational leadership. I caught up with all three of these leaders and have updated their leadership journeys.

In addition, I reworked Castellani and Hafferty's seven-clustered model of physician professionalism from their original, and at times somewhat pejorative construct, to profile additional physician leaders I greatly admire and have learned from. I hope you will be as inspired by these individuals as I have been.

SITUATIONAL LEADERSHIP

Situational leadership is built on the traits necessary for change management. Physician situational leaders are crucial to guide institutions through effective change, including medical groups, health systems, payer organizations, multinational retail enterprises entering healthcare, and publicly traded telehealth companies. They also are still needed in independent small medical practices and local communities.

Eugenie Komives, MD

In 2009, Dr. Eugenie Komives received the President's Award from the North Carolina Academy of Family Practice *"for her openness to tough discussions and the ability to facilitate dialogue with the highest level of Blue*

Cross Blue Shield management." As Vice President and Senior Medical Director of Blue Cross and Blue Shield of North Carolina, Dr. Komives used her ability to influence her colleagues to forge much more collaborative relationships between physicians in practice and the largest managed care company in the state.

After graduating from the University of Wisconsin at Madison with a degree in biochemistry in 1981, she entered Harvard Medical School and, following graduation, completed a one-year internship in internal medicine at the Beth Israel Hospital in Boston before entering the Duke Family Medicine residency program.

She subsequently spent 11 years in private practice and various part-time leadership roles with Kaiser Permanente before becoming the State Health Plan Medical Director in North Carolina in 2000. In 2005, she was promoted to Vice President and Senior Medical Director at Blue Cross Blue Shield, where she has bridged the gap between payer and provider by focusing on the quality of patient care while maintaining a sympathetic ear for those in the trenches practicing medicine.

In contrast to many physicians who leave the practice of medicine to take on positions in insurance or other non-clinical aspects of the industry, Dr. Komives has maintained an active leadership role in statewide organized medicine. She has served on the Managed Care Committee, the Quality of Care and Performance Improvement Committee, and the Accountable Care Organization Task Force of the North Carolina Medical Society, the Board of Directors for the Quality Council of North Carolina, the Board of Directors of the North Carolina Prevention Partners, and the North Carolina Academy of Family Physicians Foundation.

She has worked with the NC Medical Society's Leadership College to lead interactive group discussions on leadership skills for physicians participating in the leadership development program and written for the *NC Medical Journal* on new technologies such as electronic communication between clinicians and patients that might improve care.

While at Blue Cross and Blue Shield of North Carolina, Dr. Komives oversaw the areas of Medical and Reimbursement Policy Development, Network Quality, including Credentialing and Quality-based Network Programs, Appeals, and Accreditation. She uses her position to develop policies and programs for the largest private insurer in the state that works toward the goals of an evidence-based, high-quality, low-cost healthcare delivery system.

She developed evidence-based guidelines for payment of spinal fusion that emphasized active exercise over surgery, helped implement a Bridges to Excellence pay-for-performance program in North Carolina that helped put North Carolina physicians near the top in the nation with NCQA recognition for evidence-based medicine, and implemented the Blue Quality Physician Program with the goal of having 50% of North Carolina's primary care physicians working in a patient-centered medical home model by 2013. She helped implement a globally reimbursed payment model with a healthcare system in Gastonia, North Carolina, that incentivizes improvement through collaborative thinking as it pertains to the care experience for knee surgery that incorporates physician encounters, diagnostic testing, physical therapy services, and hospitalization into one global payment. She says:

> This is a significant step in the right direction for changing the way care is delivered, measured, and paid for in this country.

* * *

In catching up with Dr. Komives in 2021, I found her to be the same consistent physician leader who has continued to apply her leadership skills in various situations. She left BCBS of North Carolina in 2012 because she recognized a need to have more time to shepherd her children through their late high school years in preparation for college. A former clinical practice partner and friend encouraged her to re-enter a clinical practice position, and she joined Duke Primary Care as a family physician. Although she hadn't practiced medicine in 12 years, she found it was like riding a bike, recalling doing a complete neurological examination on a patient and starting from the top and moving to the feet as something that quickly came back to her as she examined the patient.

Although she was content practicing in her 0.8 FTE position, she was asked in 2014 to become the Senior Medical Director for Duke's population health management organization, and soon her clinic-to-management ratio had flipped back to about 80% management. Nonetheless, she maintained a panel of 700 patients while she and Duke Health System learned how to effectively do population health management.

She loved the opportunity to impact population health working on the provider side rather than health plan and is proud of Duke Health's success in learning what works for their patients. In 2018, Duke successfully saved Medicare $20M in the Medicare Shared Savings Program and earned $10M in savings for Duke, allowing them to pay back their investment in population health capabilities and successfully continue their ongoing journey in value-based care.

In 2019, she was asked to return to the health plan side of healthcare to become the Medical Director of WellCare's Managed Medicaid program. The North Carolina legislature had mandated the move to managed Medicaid and WellCare was one of a handful of health plans selected to stand up a product in the state.

Dr. Komives was initially recruited to this position not by the health plan directly but by Greg Griggs, Executive Vice-President of the NC Academy of Family Physicians, not WellCare. The family physicians in North Carolina wanted to make sure the Medicaid managed care organizations had excellent physician leadership.

Going live with managed Medicaid in July 2021, Dr. Komives and WellCare are learning how to pivot quickly when things are working. She continues to call providers back directly when the company gets a complaint, something she has learned goes a long way in her efforts to make sure Medicaid is "done right" in North Carolina.

Dr. Komives sees her current career trajectory as focused on the developing people in her organization, mentoring, and making sure that Medicaid managed care is executed effectively in North Carolina.

"At age 62, I'm not worried about my career," she says. "At this point it is about doing my job as best as I can do every single day, working with providers, and succession planning that will create the leaders my company needs for the ongoing work after I am no longer in this role."

SERVANT LEADERSHIP

The medical profession is built on profoundly important service to patients. Those of us privileged to take on this role may have many motivations, but the essential ethical precept upon which our privilege is based presupposes service.

Some physicians embody this servant leadership such that they rise above the day-to-day challenges we all face with humility and integrity. I witnessed Dr. Eliot Williams go to extraordinary measures to prevent a patient with Wolff-Hirschhorn syndrome from certain endotracheal intubation. Other than the nurse at the bedside and me, I doubt anyone else knows what he did.

Elliott Williams, MD

Elliott Williams, MD, says it took him a long time to even think of himself as a leader. Born the second of nine children in a working-class family with limited financial resources, he was the first in his family to go to college, which was, he says, "stepping way outside the box."

Once out of that box, Dr. Williams excelled academically, graduating cum laude from Pfeiffer College in 1983 before attending medical school at the University of North Carolina at Chapel Hill and completing his post-graduate training in anesthesiology at the University of Virginia. After staying on a year at the University of Virginia as faculty, Dr. Williams decided to enter private practice and moved his family to High Point, NC, where he joined Carolina Anesthesiology, PA, and became part of the medical staff of High Point Regional Health System where he has served in a number of leadership roles, including President of the Surgery Center Management Company, Chief of Cardiac Anesthesia, and, ultimately, a member of the hospital Board of Trustees and Chief of Staff.

Dr. Williams reflects on his leadership journey as an unintentional process that occurred out of his desire to meet the needs of those he serves in his clinical role:

> Because resources were quite limited in my family growing up, my answer to everything was to work harder. I always felt that I could overcome everyone else's advantages with hard work. I think being willing to work hard and not complain can sometimes set one apart with colleagues and employees.
>
> I think that this, along with an uncompromising desire to always be fair and honest, no matter the cost, a passion to always do my best not only for the patients but for those around me (surgeons, nurses, nurse anesthetists) and trying to always keep the big picture in focus, has caused those around me to elevate me into leadership roles.
>
> I guess until recently, I never viewed myself as a leader. My most famous saying in the OR is, 'I'm just here to lead the trucks.' However, when I was asked to be chief of staff, I had to reconsider. Subsequently, I have been much more focused on reading and learning about leadership. I feel like I am learning more and more all the time.

Dr. Williams has been honored by the nurses at High Point Regional Hospital with the Golden Stethoscope Award, given annually to the physician voted by the nurses as the most outstanding physician. He leads by example in ways that are both humble and profound.

One night, when he was the anesthesiologist on call, and the operating room was not busy, he stayed up and held in his arms all night a severely mentally disabled 85-pound woman with Wolf-Hirschhorn's syndrome hospitalized with severe pneumonia and end-stage pulmonary hypertension, in order that her exhausted family could get some much-needed rest. His actions prevented the patient from what would have certainly been endotracheal intubation or respiratory arrest and permitted the nursing staff to remain at the bedside of other patients needing their care. The patient recovered, and the medical staff and nursing staff saw one more example of a servant leader "stepping outside the box" to do what was necessary.

Dr. Williams has had an enormous influence on the culture of the medical staff of High Point Regional Hospital. The speech he gave as chief of staff at High Point Regional Health System's Foundation Endowment dinner attended by community leaders, hospital administration, and a significant number of the medical staff embodies his spirit of service and obligation, illustrates how his leadership is based on *building community, awareness, persuasion, conceptualization, foresight, stewardship, empathy, listening, commitment to growth of people,* and *healing.* He had kept a daily journal for a week writing his inner feelings, both positive and negative, and shared them at the dinner:

> I feel inadequate because I don't know what to say to this patient dying of cancer. I feel angry because yet again I have to get consent for anesthesia over the phone from the director of social services because both the parents of this 2-year-old are incarcerated. I feel nervous because I am really worried on how I am going to get this sick elderly patient through this emergency surgery. I feel uncertain because I don't know how healthcare reform will affect my ability to manage my practice and care for my patients. I feel concerned because a disproportionate number of epidurals that I do are for teenage mothers. I feel disappointment because neighboring hospitals that for years we thought were our allies have decided to become our competitors.

> However, I feel confident, for because of you, I have better equipment and technology and have been able to recruit and retain excellent colleagues. I feel relieved because I realize that you do not expect me to always know the right things to say and have all of the right answers. You expect me to do my best.

> I feel strong because the trust and confidence that you have placed in me have given me the courage to persevere. I feel excited because the excellence that you have demanded of me has caused me to strive to be better than I thought I could be. I feel proud because I know how hard the individuals here work each and every day to care for our patients and I know that you are proud of them also.

> And lastly I feel humbled to stand before such a generous and caring group.

Dr. Williams says he is passionate about "not only continuing to grow as a leader but how to help steer our hospital through challenging times.

Physicians are going to have to step forward and not only practice great medicine but also help shape the landscape of medicine. We know it from a perspective that only we can possibly know."

* * *

I caught up with Dr. Williams in July 2021 and found him to be the patient-centered servant leader I had known and admired since 1993 when we both started on staff at High Point Regional Hospital. But Dr. Williams in 2021 is much broader in his leadership focus than in the past. He has lived through the transition of the hospital from acquisition by UNC Health, then acquisition by Wake Forest Health System, an academically focused organization that itself has recently joined the large Charlotte-based Atrium Health System.

In the midst of the continued consolidation in the healthcare delivery system, Dr. William's anesthesiology group has chosen to remain independent of health system employment while continuing to serve the ongoing needs of the local medical community.

He is currently focused on nurturing awareness of the sophistication of the local High Point medical community with the sometimes tone-deaf, academically-focused Wake Forest Health System. He enjoys modeling professional behavior for the young residents now rotating through the hospital, as well as new, junior associates of his own medical group. Of the medical partners part of his group at the time he joined in 1993, all but one are either now part-time or retired.

Dr. Williams is now President of his practice group. He is proud that there have been nearly zero turnovers in the past 30 years in the practice's support staff and nurse anesthetists. During the COVID-19 pandemic outbreak in 2020, elective surgical volume dropped 80%, yet with careful management, the medical group remained financially stable and was able to retain all employees.

In reflecting upon his professional career, Dr. Williams asserts that "I haven't changed. Things that were always important to me still are: God, family, and taking good care of people." When his younger colleagues marvel at his ongoing workload, Dr. Williams reminds them of how much joy there is in the practice of medicine.

> I love medicine. If you practice it right, it is a wonderful profession. If you are good to the profession, it will be good to you. Unfortunately, some people get out of training and develop a little bit of an entitlement mentality. Coming from a blue-collar family, I have never allowed myself to get caught up in an entitlement mentality. It is just such a privilege to practice medicine.

And for the community of High Point, North Carolina, it is such a privilege to have this servant leader modeling how to remain patient- and community-focused in the midst of ongoing change.

TRANSFORMATIONAL LEADERSHIP

Sometimes the world just needs changing. The skills to do true transformational change in the healthcare industry are difficult. Those capable of doing so in large, complex institutions are very rare. Alan Kaplan has done this more than once.

Alan Kaplan, MD, MMM, FACPE, FACHE

Alan Kaplan, MD, did not set out to be the chief executive officer of a large integrated medical group. Like many pre-medical students, he had majored in biological sciences at the University of Illinois because his sights were on being a practicing physician one day. So, when he graduated from Rush Medical College in 1985, he entered an otolaryngology residency at Mayo Clinic where he had 2½ years of surgical training, prior to changing career course and going through another three-year residency in emergency medicine at Christ Hospital in Oak Lawn, Illinois.

When he entered private practice as an emergency physician in 1991, he had completed 25 years of school and medical training. He threw himself whole-heartedly into his new job while he and his wife began raising their family.

Just after three years of completing his formal medical training, he has already achieved his ultimate goal of becoming the medical director of an emergency department. Seeking additional leadership and management knowledge, he began taking courses in management through the American College of Physician Executives in the mid-90s that ultimately led to his completing a master's in medical management degree at Carnegie Mellon University in 2000.

Starting as the Chief of Emergency Services at Edward Hospital in Naperville, Illinois, in 1994, he continued toward progressively higher leadership roles with the Edward Health Services Corporation while continuing to practice emergency medicine. By 1995 he was Chief Medical Officer, and in 2004 he was promoted to Vice President, Chief Medical and Operations Officer.

A critical juncture in his career occurred in 2005 when his executive position became too large in scale and scope to continue in clinical practice, and he reluctantly made the decision to stop practicing emergency medicine.

At Edward Hospital, Dr. Kaplan's scope of responsibilities included business development, oversight of a $200 million net revenue service line that included emergency services, urgent care, corporate health, laboratory, hospitalist program, hospital-based physicians, clinical quality improvement, information systems, telecommunication, materials management, and medical staff growth and development.

In 2009, he made the career-defining decision to move his family from the urban Chicago area to Iowa, where he was employed as Vice President and Chief Medical Officer of the Iowa Health System, a fully integrated system with 19,000 employees, $2.3 billion in annual revenues, serving one of every three patients in the state of Iowa at 26 hospitals and 71 communities.

Since coming to Iowa, he is on the cusp of merging 600 physicians into a single group, developed a formal physician leadership academy, and developed and put into operation a business plan that incorporated an integrated care organization to work with both employed and independent physicians to improve quality, lower cost, and enhance the patient experience. He just completed his term as President of the American College of Physician Executives, in which he led its Board of Directors through a strategically crucial transition period for the organization. Currently, he is creating and leading an accountable care organization development team and has redesigned the quality committee of the Iowa Health System's Board.

When queried about his leadership journey, Dr. Kaplan makes it clear that this was not a planned path. "I didn't plan to be a physician executive. My goal was to be the medical director of an emergency department, I have always had a propensity to see things that needed to be done and pursue a solution. Incremental success simply led to larger administrative roles."

But having the propensity to pursue solutions permits him to have a transformative influence in the healthcare industry. "Right now, I am passionate about healthcare reform and in making sure it truly improves quality and lowers overall costs with a sharp focus on our patients and communities, as well as our physicians who are at the core of all healthcare decisions."

* * *

In 2016, Dr. Kaplan was selected to become the CEO of the University of Wisconsin Health in Madison, Wisconsin. He describes the decision to accept this role as both personally and organizationally risky, as he transitioned from being the executive vice president/chief clinical officer of UnityPoint Health, a community-oriented health system, to becoming CEO of UW Health, the academic health system affiliated with the University of

Wisconsin. He had never been CEO and had no academic health system experience. The health system was looking for a physician leader with business acumen to lead the $3.4 billion health organization that was undertaking complex initiatives, such as merging the hospital system and the faculty medical group.

Five years later, he has led the system through transformative change, sustainability during the pandemic, and is preparing the organization for its post-pandemic future. Like many organizations, UW Health implemented telehealth visits to permit ongoing access for patients during quarantine. But unlike other organizations where telehealth is diminishing, the organization's virtual-care visits continue to increase.

He believes the added turmoil of the pandemic has intensified the disruption to such that it is time to seize the opportunities to eliminate the burden of administrative waste and other health system barriers to improvement.[1] He states he remains "motivated by the desire to build things. I thrive on good strategic planning with goals, accountabilities, resources, timelines, and oversight to bring strategy to reality." He leads by taking the organization to "where they haven't gone before."[2]

NOSTALGIC LEADERSHIP (TRADITIONAL)

When Hafferty and Castellani defined their professional clusters in 2010,[3] they identified the most dominant cluster to be the nostalgic cluster, defined as the locus of traditional medical leaders in academic medicine, medical societies and trade organizations, and publications, focused on preserving physician autonomy and fighting the commercialization of medicine.

A decade later, this cluster cannot be defined by these previous goals. Much of the national leadership is forward-focused rather than nostalgic, recognizing the limitations of fee-for-service medicine and focused upon redesigning physician leadership in new models of healthcare delivery that improved patient outcomes.

Jerry Penso, MD, MBA

When Jerry Penso began his professional career, he thought he would be a practicing family physician his whole life. He practiced as part of an 80-person independent medical practice in San Diego, California, and truly enjoyed his broad practice that ranged from pre-natal visits to surgical assisting, medical care across care settings, end-of-life care, and everything in between. But life has a way of not turning out as planned. When his medical practice experienced some financial instability, it became part of a health system that had cultural expectations for every physician to take part in committees and governance. He was assigned to the Pharmacy and Therapeutics Committee, which ended up changing his life course.

At the time, his medical group was in a capitated model, taking risk on pharmacy but losing money on that part of their business. When the committee chairman had a scheduling conflict, Dr. Penso was asked to lead the committee one day. He agreed to do so after the chairman said he would create his "overhead slides" for the meeting for him ahead of time.

The meeting went well, and Dr. Penso received positive feedback, for which he was rewarded with more work and new responsibilities. He became chair of the committee and serendipitously discovered the medical group was receiving information about drug utilization from the health plan on floppy disks that had not been analyzed. He dug into the data and began presenting the information to the clinicians, who liked the feedback and insights the data provided. He considers this his first foray into population health management methodologies, and it launched his career in an entirely different direction.

From the position of losing money on pharmacy risk, Dr. Penso designed and implemented a program for his medical group that turned profitable, and then moved on to more comprehensive program development for quality improvement. He was selected to be part of the inaugural class of the California Health Foundation's physician leadership development program, where he had an 18-month deep exposure into healthcare system improvement, including personal leadership coaching, healthcare policy exposure, principles of business didactics, and the teaching on quality improvement from Dr. Brent James, a physician pioneer in health system quality improvement from Intermountain Healthcare in Utah. Dr. Penso considers Dr. James a major mentor in his own leadership journey.

After his exposure to James' methodology, Dr. Penso wanted to apply the methodology in his own health system. He left the medical group's medical practice and entered a position that was created for him at the health system level, funded by the system's two medical groups and IPA, to develop a quality improvement program for the medical groups.

Taking advantage of the new California pay-for-performance incentive program, Dr. Penso built a quality program that ranked first in the state. The medical group loved the positive financial incentives and took pride in their quality performance, and patients had a better experience and improved outcomes.

He was then asked to take on quality improvement at the state level, chairing the board of the Integrated Healthcare Association that administered the P4P program that his group had been so successful in. His medical group permitted him to take time off to go through an executive MBA program, as he wanted deeper training and experience in business processes.

Dr. Penso believes in learning from others. He became actively involved in AMGA (American Medical Group Association), where he met other medical group leaders from around the country and learned from the cultural sharing and collaboration that is the core of AMGA.

AMGA asked him to join their executive team and run their national quality program. He became AMGA's first chief medical officer and organized and led two national quality campaigns, *Pressure Up, Pressure Down,* and *Together to Goal,* which created national processes to improve blood pressure control and diabetes control. The PUPD initiative resulted in a half-million patients across the nation getting their blood pressure in control through the collaborative learning initiatives of the program.

In 2017, when Don Fisher, AMGA's CEO of 35 years, died, AMGA mounted an extensive national search and selected Dr. Penso to be the CEO. He has focused his energies as CEO on moving the AMGA culture from a "family-run business" type culture to a professional culture. His goal is to make the trade association's mission of helping medical groups thrive adequately robust and future-oriented to meet the memberships' needs for the rapidly changing healthcare delivery system. Underlying the entire arc of his professional career, healthcare improvement remains his north star.

ENTREPRENEURIAL LEADERSHIP (INNOVATION)

Entrepreneurs are risk-takers. They assume the risks of a business or enterprise and use innovation as the currency by which they succeed. Innovation is based on the ability to create something new through the use of imagination. In general, physicians have not been selected or trained for creativity. Yet, much of the progress of medicine has occurred out of the creativity of physician entrepreneurs who identify ways to improve healthcare delivery and are willing to disrupt the *status quo* to drive needed change.

Jesse James, MD, MBA

Not all men named Jesse James are outlaws. Jesse Cimarron James is the fourth Jesse James in his family, with Jr. and III serving as law enforcement officers. But Jesse James IV has a different claim to fame: He is a serial entrepreneur.

Dr. Jesse James is the Chief Medical Officer for CHESS Health Solutions, a population health management company founded in 2013 by the shareholders of Cornerstone Healthcare. His journey to this place and position has been built on a life story filled with entrepreneurial paths, turning here, turning there, but always turning to a place where he can build something new and meaningful.

He is the third son of six children, born in Chicago to a dynamic power couple: his mother, an elementary and high school English teacher, and his father, an activist minister. His family moved to Atlanta when his father became director of admissions at Morehouse University. Dr. James calls Atlanta a big city of small-town folks, where the public schools he attended were excellent and the teachers were equal parts disciplinarians and role models who loved and took pride in their students. He loved science. In fourth grade, he read his entire biology textbook the first weekend.

Dr. James attended Florida A&M, a historically black university, majored in science, and planned to pursue a PhD in cardiovascular physiology. Although surrounded by pre-med students in his classes, he wasn't interested in a medical career; he wanted basic science. During a summer internship with a cardiologist at Yale his junior year, he helped the professor set up the lab from scratch, as he had just moved from UCSD to Yale. He also was able to set up his own experiments on viral transduction to reduce ischemic to myocytes. "That building and ordering and setting up appealed a lot to me from my entrepreneurial spirit," James says.

That summer also changed his view of his career path, when the professor took him on rounds in the hospital, took him to the cath lab, showed him the results of echocardiograms and nuclear studies, and then helped him get his adenovirus vectors to infect the myocytes without too many dying before his results could be measured, ordering and building the ischemic chamber. He was now sold on the combination of clinical and scientific careers. He immediately began practicing for the MCAT, although he still was divided between a pure basic science career or a clinical one.

Dr. James says he had an epiphany when he saw a group of students taking up a collection for a dog that needed surgery, and he was reminded of all the people who didn't have access to care due to health insurance. He decided he would pursue a medical career and focus on solving the larger problems in healthcare delivery. "This was before the ACA had passed. Greater than 15% of the population didn't have health insurance. They were no better off than that dog, and I knew I wanted to do something about that," he says.

He applied to only two medical schools, the Medical College of Georgia and Yale. He decided to go north to New Haven and says he loved his first two years of basic science in medical school but really missed the easy-going friendliness of southern culture. So, by the time he began his third-year clerkships, he knew he wanted to come back south.

His residency advisor recommended the "southern alternatives of either UPenn or Johns Hopkins," but Dr. James wanted to come back to the real south. He chose to pursue internal medicine at the University of North Carolina at Chapel Hill, thinking he would then pursue cardiology.

Before he went south, he decided to get his MBA. He wanted to have an impact on the big, deep issues of healthcare delivery. Dr. James found the MBA to be the hardest part of medical school. Having had no previous exposure to such concepts as financial accounting, net present value, how to decide on a project, how to take risks, were entirely new ways of thinking. He muses:

> The concept in business that you should learn how to take on risks and being willing to fail was a whole new way for the young scientist to think. Medicine likes precision and we like success. Learning how to fail and learning from failure are just not values we are comfortable with in medicine.

Dr. James unreservedly talks about his Christian faith, as it influences how he has pursued his professional life:

> I remember the parable of the 10 talents. One of the servants buried in the ground the coins his master had asked him to steward because he didn't want to take a risk. We are called in life to take risks. There is both a Christian value and a business value to take on risk smartly, so you are called to sometimes fail. If you are always succeeding, you are burying your talents in the ground. The parable is pushing you to use what you got.

He chose UNC-Chapel Hill over residency in Chicago (too cold!) and Duke because he was attracted to the preventative medicine program at UNC and its social medicine department. He had found about the program online and realized, "these are my people. I didn't even know social medicine was a thing. I read Dr. Jon Oberlander's books; I was a huge fan. This department was thinking the same thoughts and doing the same things I wanted to do and doing it better than I ever could have. That's providence for me."

He liked UNC's culture. "As a state hospital, there was no VIP; everybody got great care, regardless of social class or status." He stayed five years, completing both an internal medicine and preventative medicine residency. "The heart, the brains, the faith you need to practice were all there. I loved what I learned there. There were great professors of medicine who took their mission to the community seriously."

At the end of the residency, he was looking at cardiology fellowships for a next career step, but it was the summer of the passage of the Affordable Care Act. He was working in a boutique policy firm called Avalere in Washington DC, briefing the team on the transcripts from the Senate Finance Committee and realized how much he was loving this work. "There was so much opportunity to change healthcare in ways that had not previously been possible." He was excited about ACA, being in DC, and thinking about policy.

He was also very much influenced by healthcare events in his own family. His father was in a hospital in Chicago to prepare for a cholecystectomy the next day. He had a middle cerebral artery stroke that the staff did not recognize until it was too late to give him TPA and open up the clotted artery and preserve brain tissue. He had another stroke when a coumadin dose was not changed with his INR out at 14 seconds.

Dr. James says he needed to get out of training and into a paying job, as his family had been sacrificing for the sake of his training, and it was time to give back: "It was time to grow up and work and do more."

He took a job with Inovalon, the largest outsourced HEDIS vendor, where he got to work with Cary Sennett, the Chief Medical Officer. He remembers leadership advice Dr. Sennett gave him, which he takes to heart to this day: "Jesse, I haven't gotten it all figured out."

James describes how Sennet's humility impacted his view of what good leadership looked like: "He was a pillar in the industry I wanted to work with, but he is humbly telling me 'I am going to get some things wrong. I am going to get some things right. I want you to feel empowered to correct me when it is needed.' I thought that was very humble and the type of leadership I wanted to mirror."

At Inovalon, Dr. James built out algorithms for fraud, waste, and abuse in Medicare Advantage billing. Then he started working on a predictive model for the Medicare Advantage stars quality program in the first year the program was rolled out by CMS. He learned to admire the discipline around software coding. He led a team. He learned to shift deeply into data analysis and development.

Then he joined Farzad Mostashiri at the Office of the National Coordinator for Health Information as part of the Obama administration in the middle of the meaningful use development policies. He found the team that built out the quality measures for CMS to be a very small entrepreneurial team. He built quality measures for CMS collaborating EMR vendors to build measures that could be usefully measured at the population level.

After his time at ONC, he joined the private company Evolent where he was tasked with finding the sequel based coding logic to digitize chronic disease reduction. He built out predictive models for outcomes to use those models to stratify patients in the cost reduction program for care management. He started with a chronic disease reduction program and learned to build something that would scale. He learned how to grow a team and hire, grow, organize, and work remotely together.

As Evolent grew, Dr. James had to expand his own role from being the medical director who knew every piece of code and every piece of logic to one who had to manage teams acquired, remote, and culturally different than the small in-person shop he had when Evolent was small.

But Dr. James knew he liked the steep part of the entrepreneurial curve. So, his next move was to come to CHESS, as Chief Medical Officer, to begin the team building and innovation all over again. He is enjoying being closer to the clinical work with a pharmacy team and care management team. He is ready to grow something again.

He reflects on leadership as it relates to his education and career path. "You learn leadership in business school, but not in medical school. In medicine, you learn leadership by seeing attending physicians and colleagues you want to be like and others you absolutely don't."

He believes having a more former leadership development process in medicine would not be a bad thing.

> I believe I am doing a good job as a leader when I step in when they need it and step back when they do not so they can shine. I think a good attending or master clinician can teach them about practice without getting too involved and letting that physician practice and develop their own style. In the OR, the most senior attendings were the most relaxed.

He believes this is servant leadership: leading but also serving the team.

He reflects that his toughest times as a leader have been when he has had to think through termination and remediation. He doesn't believe, in medicine, we train well to do that. We have difficulty with the challenges of navigating tolerance versus boundaries of performance to protect teams. "There is a responsibility as a leader to be aggressive to stop misbehavior as early as possible."

Despite these hard leadership challenges, Dr. James is an optimist, "In summary, I've been able to do my dream job, even when I didn't have it all dreamed out. It is a blessing every day."

ACADEMIC LEADERSHIP (TEACHING)

Physician teachers currently have many challenges. Medical education funding sources still funnel most medical education to acute hospital settings. Most academicians must support themselves with clinical work or research grants that limit their time and focus on teaching. In general, compensation lags those in private practice with whom they must compete for patients. Cultural and gender diversity remains limited in academic medical settings, with ongoing challenges for women and racial and cultural minority physicians to attain equivalent compensation, funding, and tenure.

Dekarlos Dial, DPM

Dr. Dekarlos Dial grew up in a large extended family in Bessemer, Alabama, where a strong work ethic and entrepreneurial culture-infused his day-to-day experience. His blue-collar family valued work and faith, and he says he was raised by the extended community comprising his parents, grandparents, and church community.

Around age 10 or 11, he learned from his grandfather that he should have thought to cut the unmown grass of an elderly neighbor on his own, and not expect to be paid, because he would be awarded in other ways. He says he most definitely was awarded, favored by this elderly woman until the day she died.

Dr. Dial was the first person in his family to go to college. He majored in biology and pre-med at Talladega College, a private liberal arts, historically black college about an hour from his home. He had the opportunity to shadow Dr. David Robinson, a podiatrist in Birmingham, as an undergraduate, and immediately determined he wanted to become a podiatrist. He admired the attention Dr. Robinson paid to his patients and his overall attention to their care. He noticed a refrigerator full of homemade desserts from grateful patients and the deep physician-patient relationship Dr. Robison developed with his patients.

Following in his mentor's footsteps, Dr. Dial entered the Ohio College of Podiatric Medicine in Cleveland. After completing the degree, he moved to Pittsburgh, Pennsylvania, to do a three-year foot and ankle fellowship at the University of Pittsburgh. He became the first podiatry resident to be accepted and trained in a reconstructive foot and ankle fellowship in the department of orthopedic surgery at UPMC.

After he and his wife, Tasha, a pediatrician, completed their training at UPMC, Dr. Dial began focusing his job search on academic positions. Academic centers such as Duke and UPMC interested him. However, he ultimately chose to join a private multispecialty medical group, Cornerstone Healthcare, in High Point, North Carolina, because he liked its innovative culture.

When he made this decision, his faculty mentors at UPMC told him he was "wasting" his career by entering practice in a community they had never heard of, not affiliated with a medical school. But Dr. Dial thrived as a leader in private practice. Over the next 15 years, he was elected to the Board of Directors of Cornerstone, then to the Board of Directors of CHESS, a population health management company. He served as Chief of Surgery at Thomasville Hospital, part of the Novant Health system, President of the NC Foot and Ankle Society, President of the Save-a-leg-and-save-a-life Foundation, and Scientific and Academic Chair of the state podiatry society, all the while practicing reconstructive foot and ankle medicine full time and parenting a son and a daughter.

However, the urge to teach as part of an academic practice never left him. While at Cornerstone, he served as an adjunct faculty at Wake Forest School of Medicine in the newly formed podiatric residency program. After Cornerstone was acquired by Wake Forest Health System, Dr. Dial moved full-time into an academic role at Wake Forest, as assistant professor and program director for the podiatric residency program.

His days now begin at 5 am, when he reads for 45 minutes, then attends case conferences from 6:00 am to 7:30, filling the rest of his days with his academic roles in the clinic, the operating room, research, grand rounds, other teaching conferences, and day-to-day teaching of residents. He loves the cross-specialty collaborative relationships he has engendered with vascular surgery and, most of all, teaching.

He says he gets up every day absolutely loving what he does. "What I enjoy most is teaching residents the really important parts of taking care of patients. I want them to know how to talk to patients and get to know them as people, how to take time with them."

Dr. Dial states he prioritizes first faith, then family, and thirdly, podiatry. Somehow, he does this while showing medical learners what professionalism is really all about.

LIFESTYLE LEADERSHIP (PHYSICIAN WELLNESS)

In the past, physicians who placed strong values on achieving a work-life balance between their time at work and family, spiritual, personal health needs or outside interests were encouraged to keep quiet about it, as the dominant expectation was physician work was to supersede all other priorities. With the recognition of the epidemic of physician burnout, this stance is no longer tolerated, and numerous physicians are leading in redefining the work-life balance necessary for physician healthiness.

Jennifer Byrne, MD, PHD

Dr. Jennie Byrne is a musician. At a young age, she played the violin, then switched to bassoon in middle school when someone declared she would not be able to play it. Play it, she did, and she went to the University of Pennsylvania as a performance major playing the bassoon. She also is a scientist, earning a PhD from New York University in 2003, one year before receiving her MD from NYU.

Dr. Byrne believes this binary aspect of her experience is rooted in her lifelong ability to "fall in between two worlds and translate between them" and is crucial in understanding her leadership approach.

Her dual worldview developed in the small central Pennsylvania community where she grew up. Her family was affluent, but she went to public schools where the majority of the students were impoverished. Only 9% of her high school class went to college. In high school, she found recognition as a musician but also read voraciously and loved math and science. Dr. Byrne says, "I wasn't one of those kids who knew they wanted to grow up and be a doctor." Despite the fact that her maternal grandfather was a pediatrician and her maternal grandmother was a chemist in the 1930s, her family did not push her toward a STEM-tracked life path. She always enjoyed working. Beginning with the paper route she had at age 14 onward, she always worked multiple jobs, exposing her to many different types of people along the way.

Feeling constrained in the small town where she grew up, Dr. Byrne went to Paris for a college semester, then talked her parents into letting her stay for a year until she ran out of money. In Paris, she took a 100% humanities-based course load, taught entirely in French. But when she returned to UPenn, she took a neuroscience course in brain and behavior, which completely changed her life trajectory. She worked in a research lab with Dr. Irwin Lucki, a supportive mentor who encouraged her to become an MD-PhD.

The bassoon-playing fine arts performance major ended up graduating with a Bachelor of Arts in the Biological Basis of Behavior and French in 1995.

After college, she got a research job at the Veteran's Hospital West Haven, Connecticut, and spent the year completing preparing for the MCAT. She began her combined MD-PhD program in 1997 at New York University, completing a basic science PhD over the course of five years in Multielectrode Neurophysiology of Attention.

Dr. Byrne felt pulled toward clinical work, looking at both neurology and psychiatry residency programs and ultimately deciding on psychiatry because she "liked the quirkiness of its culture compared to the more buttoned-up culture of neurology." Although she continued to research in residency on cognitive deficits in schizophrenia and functional MRI imaging, she was exposed to entirely new (non-biological) ways of thinking.

Her four-year psychiatry resident at Mount Sinai in New York included a recommendation that she undergo psychotherapy as part of the experience necessary to provide this service to patients as a physician. Initially skeptical, she found this experience transformative, opening her eyes to a healthier self-awareness that has allowed her to design a career built for resiliency and personal health while also taking care of others.

This deeper self-awareness allowed her to realize the career path she was being encouraged to pursue as a physician-scientist was not the life path she wanted to pursue. She was "getting fed up with academia," including its unrealistic expectations of years of the low salary in science research. She had a baby at this time and did not believe the academic path of a $17,000 a year post-doc fellowship salary while living in New York City was practical or desirable. So, she and her growing family made a "leap of faith" move to North Carolina. Here, she saw varied and innovative career opportunities, taking a job as a psychiatrist for Doctors Making Housecalls for two years.

In 2010, Dr. Byrne had an entrepreneurial itch and started up her own private psychiatry practice from scratch: Cognitive Psychiatry of Chapel Hill. The practice performed outpatient evaluation, psychopharmacology, psychotherapy, and substance use disorder treatment across the lifespan. She had to construct and implement a business model, including the documentation, communications, billing, technology, marketing, and recruiting strategies, ultimately growing the practice to more than 600 patients in the nine years she owned it. "I did it all: I was the CEO, COO, CFO, receptionist, interior decorator, social media marketer, and occasional janitor!"

Simultaneously, she worked for Community Care of North Carolina (CCNC), an organization focused on serving 1.7 million Medicaid patients and 6,000 providers in North Carolina who provided care for them. The experience of moving between the two worlds of her private cash-paying patients and the work she was doing for Medicaid patients at CCNC felt as natural as moving between the fine arts and science, and her early experience in the worlds of affluence intermixed with poverty.

Over the next 10 years, her Medicaid responsibilities grew, as she served as Deputy Chief Medical Officer and Behavioral Health Leader for CCNC. She ultimately sold her private practice in 2019. At CCNC she created the Medicaid Integrated Medial Homes strategy, leading to a reduction in hospital admission by 27% and readmissions by 59%. She designed and implemented the federal CMS Practice Transformation Network collaborative and developed multiple educational programs and behavioral health practice toolkits for medical homes and case managers, improving provider satisfaction while reducing the need for specialty referrals in the community.

The political winds in North Carolina changed when the state legislature chose managed Medicaid as a new delivery model. Dr. Byrne knew CCNC would have a less impactful position in Medicaid, so she took a role as Chief Behavioral Health Officer at Caremore Health, the healthcare delivery system renowned for its remarkable value-based models of care for Medicare Advantage patients.

At Caremore, she transformed the national behavioral health strategy and was quickly promoted to be a Vice President of Clinical Excellence for the entire clinical organization. She managed a team of six senior physician leaders and led a clinical practice team of 50 behavioral health clinicians. She also served as a mentor and coach for six other physician leaders and designed and executed high-yield clinical care pathways and didactic programming for 400 generalist and specialist clinicians. She learned the importance of proper design for strategy to be effective, how to have difficult conversations with the physicians she led, and how to work with and coach physicians who were struggling.

In 2021, Dr. Byrne left Caremore to begin a full-time role as strategy consultant and to develop a private practice devoted entirely to physicians in need of coaching or more definitive behavioral healthcare for those in need. Her innovative practice, Constellation PLLC, is named for her ongoing desire to connect the dots between people and ideas in new and unexpected ways.

From her work at CCNC and Caremore, she observed that many physicians thrust into leadership roles often struggle due to lack of training, gaps in communication skills, or, sometimes, low emotional quotients. (EQs). She observes that many clinical leaders do not have the psychology skills needed to motivate others, and her practice is focused on providing a nuanced approach to coaching, psychotherapy, or, if needed, psychopharmacologic therapies for those in need of broader behavioral health approaches.

She offers three leadership observations for physicians.

First, she believes the idea of a mentor for women physicians is not always helpful or practical. She believes the dearth of current women role models limits the effectiveness of this leadership development strategy and believes coaching provides a more adequate scale to advance women's leadership skills.

Second, she has been exposed to the ideas of authentic leadership and believes this framework is highly effective for physician leaders. The idea of authentic leadership is to begin with the knowledge that you don't have to put on a mask when going into a work role. Bringing one's best self to work by being authentic, including showing some vulnerability, leads to stronger influence and effectiveness.

Third, taking care of oneself is an essential skill for physician leaders. Physicians are trained to work all the time, to put on a stoic mask, and sacrifice their own needs for the sake of others. But if a physician is tired, not eating well, not exercising, it will show up in reduced effectiveness. "The energy you bring to your work matters," Dr. Byrne observes. "Real vacations, sleep, exercise, healthy food matters."

In her new role as physician leader coach, she uses her keen observation skills to guide physicians to healthier, sustainable leadership.

EMPIRICAL LEADERSHIP (RESEARCH)

The importance of ongoing physician leadership in research has never been greater than during the current global pandemic. Perhaps the greatest scientific achievement thus far in the 21st century has been the deployment of highly effective vaccinations for COVID-19 within a year of the onset of the pandemic. The interplay between physician as clinician and physician as medical scientist remains crucial, especially as we face the ongoing need to manage an aging world population facing the clinical consequences of climate change and resource depletion.

David Bick, MD

If initial diagnostic tests fail, physicians may move to more tests and ultimately arrive at an accurate diagnosis and treatment plan. However, for many patients with rare diseases, this diagnostic odyssey can take years.

Dr. David Bick is one of the world's foremost precision medicine specialists. He specializes in the diagnosis and treatment of rare diseases, and he wants to fundamentally change the way clinicians practice medicine.

Rare and undiagnosed diseases have an enormous and unrecognized impact on one in 10 patients and families worldwide. Rare disease affects 20–30 million Americans, with 30% of patients waiting 5–30 years for a correct diagnosis. What's more, 5% of the pediatric population has a rare disease, accounting for 12% of admissions and 16%–28% of the total cost of care for a pediatric patient.

Although rare and undiagnosed disease touches every hospital system and every specialty, it is often overlooked as a driver of the total cost of care. More than 60% of rare disease patients receive conflicting treatments options, and these illnesses are six times more expensive to treat. More than 10% of inpatient costs come from the 2% of the population who have a rare disease.

Dr. Bick is the chief medical officer and a faculty investigator at the Hudson-Alpha Institute for Biotechnology, and the medial director of the Smith Family Clinic for Genomic Medicine, a clinic specializing in the rapid diagnosis of rare disease by incorporating whole genome sequencing technology into the diagnostic process. His journey to this world-altering medical clinic is one from a strong academic and research background.

After graduating from Cornell University in 1977, he entered George Washington University School of Medicine, then completed his post-graduate education at Yale with a pediatrics internship and residency, followed by a research fellowship at Yale in Human Genetics, completed in 1987.

Subsequently, he has held academic appointments at the University of Texas, the University of Virginia, the Medical College of Wisconsin, and the University of Alabama at Birmingham. He is an international leader in genomic medicine and has published more than 100 peer-reviewed articles, chapters, and reviews, and mentored many medical students, residents, and fellows.

He is most renowned for being part of the team at the Medical College of Wisconsin who made the first diagnosis of a rare disease in a child using genomic sequencing that resulted in a life-saving bone marrow transplant.

This technology was in its earliest development at the time, but its innovative use allowed a diagnosis and treatment plan to save the life of a dying child. This story led to the Pulitzer Prize-winning article and subsequent book *One in a Billion*, documenting this scientific and medical team's remarkable work.

The success of that pioneering work led Dr. Bick to join the HudsonAlpha Institute for Biotechnology in 2015, as the Medical College of Wisconsin determined ongoing work by the genomic medicine team was too costly and not part of the medical school's core mission. At HudsonAlpha, Dr. Bick established the Smith Family Clinic, which concentrates all of its efforts on the diagnosis of rare, undiagnosed, and often misdiagnosed diseases. He states,

> Our patients have been searching for answers for an average of more than seven years, have seen dozens of doctors, and have been misdiagnosed at least twice. To have to deal with that, on top of day-to-day living with a rare disease, is excruciating. I'm proud to be part of the team providing answers and solutions to patients and their families.

As the cost of whole-genome sequencing (WGS) continues to decrease, Dr. Bick sees a future where healthy individuals have genomic sequencing at birth, with prevention and life-planning permitting individualized medicine treatments and reduction of chronic diseases and the one in 10 of us with rare diseases have them diagnosed early.

Recently he has been attacking one of the issues that arise when more diagnoses of rare diseases are made: ensuring physicians have ready access to available treatments for these disorders. He has created a website and app freely available to physicians worldwide with a summary of current treatments of the reporting literature for nearly 700 rare genetic disorders that he regularly updates(www.rx-gene.com.)[4] and is about to launch an API for use by clinical laboratories, research laboratories, and electronic medical records systems that want to include the information in reports to provide to physicians in real-time anywhere in the world.

He will shortly be joining a team focused on deploying whole genomic as an adjunct to the routine newborn screening to search for the disorders that should be treated shortly after birth to be the most effective. He believes the use of CRISPR technology will dramatically increase the number of treatable genetic disorders. For David Bick, the future is just around the corner.

ACTIVIST LEADERSHIP (POLICY)

Activist leaders strive to bring about political and social change. Physicians who are activists are natural optimists who are able to identify the problems in the current healthcare delivery system and seek improvement via tactical changes in policy at the local, state, or national levels. Typically, their impetus for action is based upon deep-seated contempt for injustice and visionary clarity around alternative paths forward.

Kavita Patel, MD, MSHS

Dr. Kavita Patel is a Texan. She was born in Dallas and grew up in San Antonio, in a first-generation Indian-American working-class family. At times, her family experienced extreme periods of unemployment and financial insecurity. When she was accepted to college at both Stanford and the University of Texas at Austin, she worried about the financial insecurity she might face from the costs of college education, so she chose the state university, where she received a full scholarship, to the private one with only partial support.

She thrived in the intellectually rich liberal arts honors program, looking at law school as her career path. She says she "got spit right into my first experience with activism," protesting Desert Storm at the state capital with Ann Richards, "one of the great southern Democrats."

In her senior year, her thesis was focused on the use of medical experts in legal cases. Pouring through these physician testimonies at the law library led her to change her career path from law to medicine. After scrambling a bit to complete her basic science courses, she was accepted into medical school at the University of Texas.

At medical school, she felt disconnected from most of her medical school classmates, who did not have the same interests she did in the impact of poverty and culture on people's health, nor the creative energy of her liberal arts college friends. However, a small group of friends developed with similar interests, and they have remained close ever since. She got involved in the American Medical Student Association (AMSA) and realized its power to impact important social issues in healthcare. She says she felt like she had finally "met my people."

After her third year of medical school, she was elected to be the national President of AMSA. She remembers her father panicked when she told him this would involve a year out of school, running a national organization, but her dean wrote a letter to her parents and explained its importance, and her family accepted the decision.

The year at AMSA was life-changing. She was effectively a CEO of a national organization with staff and resources and was able to direct the organization and impact social issues, including discounts on textbooks for medical students and advocacy for the need for diversity in medical school. Then, she returned to complete medical school, thinking seriously about surgery, but skeptical of the pyramid-type advancement structures in surgical residency where she saw no women had ever survived the residency program through all five program years.

She opted for internal medicine, attracted to the complex patients and long-term impact that can occur with longitudinal relationships, and decided, based on her national experience in AMSA, to leave Texas. She matched into the primary care tract in a medical residency in Portland, Oregon, drawn to the "real world" of ambulatory care rather than the overly structured hospital setting. She says she "faded from activism" at this time because she wanted to focus on becoming a great doctor and threw herself completely into her role as a physician, working very, very hard to be great at what she did. She became Chief Resident.

But then her "activism gene" kicked in again and she decided a public health degree would allow her to have an impact beyond her ongoing work as a clinician. She still worried about the costs of another degree, so she looked around for options that would not cost $40,000. She finally got to California, when she was awarded a Robert Wood Johnson Clinical Scholars Fellowship and matched at UCLA. This Robert Wood Johnson fellowship has been the training ground for many of the United States' great public policy medical leaders.

She focused on the work clinicians did in non-patient care that did not add value and pandemic preparedness. She received a professorship at UCLA and was awarded a grant by the RAND Corporation and practiced medicine two days a week. She states the job did not excite her, except when she was able to take her research and translate it to policy makers. She was impacted by a colleague who stated she needed to have a job that she woke up and loved every day. This led to her being offered a job with Senator Ted Kennedy.

She took a risk and took the job and moved to Washington, DC. Her boyfriend, a specialist in medical informatics, took a risk, too. They moved to the nation's capital and were married, and her life took an entirely different trajectory. She worked for years for Senator Kennedy, preparing pieces of legislation on cancer, quality of care, a children's disease registry, implementing some of the earliest genetic disease registry policies now common in most states. She got up every day and was excited for the work she was doing and the team she was part of. She learned title does not matter, *per se* — although for women, it may matter more — but the team is crucial. She explains, "Whenever I have failed in my career, which is often, it is because I failed to pay enough attention to the team."

She worked with Senator Kennedy until his glioblastoma diagnosis. After his death, she planned to return to California, where she had "family and connections and people who valued me" when she was asked to be part of Barack Obama's White House healthcare team.

In retrospect, she says, she did not realize how hard a job it was to do. She was young and working on one of the most important pieces of legislation in our lifetimes, the Affordable Care Act, but she found this team harder to work with due to its lack of cohesiveness and the personal ambitions of many of the team members. She left the White House team without securing a job and was feeling very burned out.

She says in retrospect, she was probably clinically depressed. She had not been able to practice medicine while working in the Senate or White House due to policy around conflict of interest. She yearned to get back into the practice of medicine. She had worked with the dean at Johns Hopkins on healthcare reform and was able to get started in a community-based clinic in Washington, DC affiliated with Johns Hopkins.

Mark McClellan, the administrator for the Centers for Medicare & Medicaid Services during the George W. Bush administration, asked her to work with him at the Brookings Institution. For the past 10 years, she has "managed to thread the needle with practice and policy" through the Obama, Trump, and Biden administrations. She is currently completing her second term as a member of the Physician-focused Payment Technical Advisory Committee (PTAC) that advised the Secretary of Health and Human Services on physician-focused alternative payment models.

She had a brief stint as a hospital executive at Hopkins. She calls it "one of her failures" because she was attracted to the title but not the work. "In my midlife, I have learned I just need to get up and be happy" with what I am going to work on. "I have always been part of big organizations and lead organizations, but these days I find I can be more effective in my own voice."

Dr. Patel says that pain points in her career have often resulted from her trait as a "people pleaser." "I didn't know how to say 'no' earlier in life. I would over commit and under deliver. It took me doing this serially and have people disappointed to learn."

She moved from one day a week in clinic and four days a week at Brookings to gradually reversing it such that she was working four days in the clinic and finding she was trying so hard to meet her patients' needs and the policy expectations simultaneously that she just couldn't get the job done. She says she didn't know how to ask for help. She learned she was afraid to express concerns in a constructive way sometimes. She always had respect for authority and found that when older people in positions of authority on the team stated something she disagreed with, she didn't know how to disagree constructively and would stay quiet, learning that sometimes led to bad consequences she had foreseen but not stopped.

In performance reviews, this was interpreted as not being strategic enough in her thinking. "I've had to learn how to both shut up and speak up at the right times in the right ways." She says, "another failure is that I have always tried to choose a path when I'm swimming upstream. I always have a feeling that the grass is greener, that I'm left out professionally."

These days, she is more clinically focused and has learned to be a public voice for policy improvement from the voice of a clinician seeing an underserved population of patients in urban Washington. "You read a bio, including mine, and you see a lot of pizzazz and jazz, but a lot of pain goes into that." That pain and pizzazz infused authenticity into her clinical and advocacy voice, heard nationwide as a commentator on MSNBC.

During the 2020 COVID pandemic, Dr. Patel threw herself into the clinical realm nearly full time, but she remains a voice of activism by accepting a contract with MSNBC as a commentator. She also regularly tweets and blogs on health policy and continues to contribute to research and articles at Brookings. She has learned how to use the media as an authentic and passionate physician advocating for healthcare policy that is people-focused and just. Follow her @kavitapmd.

TACTICAL LEADERSHIP

Hafferty and Castellani describe a cluster of medical professionals as "unreflective," focused mostly on the day-to-day work that typifies patient care. The term "unreflective" is unfortunate and pejorative and does not adequately define the group of clinician leaders who are providing the majority of the heavy lifting of patient care management and improvement on an ongoing basis. Tactical leaders perform the core day-to-day operational work necessary for health system improvement and serve as the crucial leaders keeping our medical groups, hospitals, clinics, operating rooms, and health systems running.

Elisabeth Stambaugh, MD, MMM

Dr. Elisabeth Stambaugh still wonders how she ended up here. She is Chief Medical Officer of the Wake Forest Health Network, an integrated health delivery system affiliated with the Wake Forest University school of medicine and Atrium Health system. She says if she were able to go back and tell her 30-year-old self what she was doing now, she would be totally astonished. "I wanted to be a doctor. I wanted to be an ob-gyn. I liked the surgical aspects of the specialty and was good at it. I became a local expert in pelvic reconstructive surgery. And I was happy."

As she took on her first healthcare leadership roles early in her career, she moved up the ladder from Ob-Gyn Section Chief to Medical Staff Executive Committee, and then to Chief of the Medical Staff of High Point Regional Health System where she practiced medicine. It took Dr. Greg Taylor, Chief Medical Officer of the hospital, to point out to her that she was, in fact, a leader, and a very good one. Before this, she thought she rose into these positions "*because I was next.*" She found she enjoyed the roles and got feedback that she was good at it. She began to take courses on leadership and was able to work with an executive coach. She observed other physician leaders in the community and learned from them.

She also found she was looking for a change both personally and professionally. She felt the pressure of "trying to be everything for everyone." She and her husband were the parents of three small children, with many of the primary childrearing responsibilities falling predominantly on her. She continued to take active ob-gyn call every four nights, practice full time, and simultaneously hold major leadership roles at the hospital.

Feeling "it was just too much," Dr. Stambaugh met with her ob-gyn practice group to negotiate refocused medical practice such that she would back off from obstetrics but continue her more manageable gynecological practice. She started the meeting saying, "I don't want to do this to you, I want to figure this out with you." What happened next, she says, was one of the ugliest moments of her career. One of her partners said, "How dare you, we brought you here." Another said, "I didn't tell you to have three kids." That partner also had three children, but had a wife who stayed at home full time. He warned her about "competing interests" related to her hospital leadership role, although he himself had previously held that role and had encouraged her to participate in hospital leadership. At this juncture in her career, trying to enlist her colleagues to help her solve her dilemma did not work.

Shortly afterward, Dr. Greg Taylor asked her to take a walk. He was moving on to another position and asked her to apply for his job. She says it had never really occurred to her that physician leadership could in and of itself be a full-time job. She chose not to apply for the position at that time, but began thinking about her career trajectory differently. She realized that the number of physicians who wanted to do leadership work and were good at it was small.

Her ob-gyn practice had joined the large community multispecialty group Cornerstone Healthcare. She moved from clinical service line leader to half-time Senior Medical Director, and subsequently took on the full-time role of Chief Medical Officer at Cornerstone Healthcare. This gradual movement from part-time to a full-time leadership role allowed her to confirm that was the direction she wanted to go and reassure her husband's misgivings, who worried she would regret moving to a full-time leadership position.

It was a tumultuous time at Cornerstone when Dr. Stambaugh became full-time CMO. Cornerstone had been a pioneer in the move from volume to value, but the group experienced significant financial instability as a result of local market forces, such as payers unwilling to partner in value-based contracts and local hospitals competing with independent groups by hiring physicians at higher compensation rates based on fee-for-service high utilization business models.

She describes this time as a rocky road, dealing with the good and bad, building some very progressive programs, interacting with disgruntled and sometimes disruptive physicians, dealing with financial instability when a large number of specialist physicians left the group to become employees of the hospital. But she quickly honed her skills in managing physician performance, by leading from a position of advocacy, empathy, and accountability.

But Dr. Stambaugh says the most difficult time of her career was a bit later, after Cornerstone joined Wake Forest Health System. The way she looks at her job is as a translator, translating business rationale and strategy to physicians, listening to physicians' concerns, and making those concerns understood by system leaders. But the first nine months after Cornerstone joined Wake Forest, she found this very hard to do, as "we were constantly told that the Cornerstone leadership didn't know what we were doing and didn't know how to run practices."

Outside consultants were brought in to reduce expenses, and rapidly eliminated much of the value-based infrastructure Cornerstone had built. But she survived this time as a leader, and ultimately was promoted to Chief Medical

Officer of the entire Wake Forest Health Network, where she is a leader in the health system's own cultural journey.

She enjoys her role as "chief translator," advocating for the front-line physician and gently nudging the Wake Forest network back to a sustainable value-based delivery system culture. She has stopped stating that her leadership position was "accidental," realizing that women often say that when really it was a recognition of effectiveness that got them in a position to lead in the first place. She continues to practice gynecology and feels it is very important to do so. She believes it keeps her grounded as a health system leader.

Dr. Stambaugh has been recruited for other leadership positions but chooses for now to remain in her current role. So long as she can keep being the advocate for physicians and for value-based healthcare, for transitioning to a world that is focused on keeping people out of the emergency room, not filling the hospital.

She decided she can make a bigger difference being in the system, not outside of it. She does not know what the future will hold, but she is confident she will continue to seek roles where she can be an advocate for value-based care and physician well-being. She says her overall philosophy is "every single thing that comes across her desk and every single decision she makes is about trying to do the right thing: patients first, then providers, then the organization."

She feels she can take complex information, make quick decisions, and adjust when subsequent information necessitates a change in course. "It's not about always doing everything right, but always trying to do the right thing." She has learned that she needs to lead by giving information, allowing people time to synthesize the information, and coming to their own decision.

She states that titles used to mean more to her than they do now. Now it is about the effectiveness and integrity of work she does in her daily job. In 10 years, she says, her daily work will still need to be about advocacy. She has learned to listen to understand, not to respond. She has also learned to make difficult decisions. "As a leader, if you aren't willing to make a difficult decision, then that means someone else will have to make that decision. And that's not fair either."

She also has learned to be self-aware of how her gender impacts her ability to lead effectively.

It is a fundamental truth that we still live in a world where the division of labor is uneven. At work, we also still have to work to lean in, in daily professional life to make sure our voices are heard, to understand that a strong woman leaders is often viewed as a bitch, while a strong male leader would never be viewed in that way. The key is to be an effective leader, and we make incremental progress through our effectiveness every day.

When sexism is apparent, she calls it out. But often, it is insidious. Relying on the tactic effective women leaders have used for ages, she simply leads with competence and effectiveness. Accidentally a leader or not, her strategy works.

STRATEGIC LEADERSHIP

Scott Ransom, DO, MPH, MBA

"With that handwriting, young man, you are either going to end up being a high school dropout or a doctor," Scott Ransom's second-grade teacher told him. He wasn't sure what a high school dropout was at the time, but it didn't sound good. However, the idea of becoming a doctor was exciting. He imagined himself a solo, small-town family doctor, much like the one in his Washington state hometown.

So, perhaps his poor penmanship began a multifaceted professional journey that included becoming an academic physician, NIH and NSF funded researcher, prolific author, tenured professor, health system executive, medical school president, university system vice chancellor for health affairs, and now a national leader in healthcare strategy.

From his small-town roots, he went off to Pacific Lutheran University, where he majored in chemistry. The degree choice was the result of his pre-med advisor, a chemistry professor, telling him that chemistry was the degree that the best pre-medical students pursued. After college, he went on to the same medical school as his doctor, Kansas City University, planning on a career in family medicine with the intent of returning to his community to become the small town's doctor.

He enjoyed medical school and was fully focused on becoming that small-town doctor until he delivered his first baby. He recalls, "it was like fireworks shooting off in my head"! Dr. Ransom then knew, "I have to do this," and made the change to obstetrics.

He loved his obstetrics and gynecology residency at Beaumont's Hospital in Dearborn, Michigan, where he trained at the large community hospital as well as the closely affiliated University of Michigan Hospital. While he loved clinical ob-gyn, especially working with complicated patients, he began conducting cost-effectiveness analysis research and became hooked. He won several hospital, state, and national prizes for research and quickly developed a passion for continuing research into his post-residency career.

His interest in improving care models and better understanding healthcare delivery systems accelerated when he became exposed to the business aspects of medicine as a chief resident. He participated in several meetings where the processes and nuances of supply chain management, billing and coding, patient throughput, and clinical labor were discussed, and reflected that "I have to be a part of that." As a chief resident, he saw the profound impact of the business of medicine on clinical practice and added another complement to his career trajectory.

His first post-residency job was as a faculty member at the Wayne State University School of Medicine and Detroit Medical Center, where he delivered babies, did surgery, conducted research, wrote dozens of articles, began writing and editing books, and worked with students and residents. He simultaneously served in several administrative roles with the health system that began his management journey.

His administrative career progressed rapidly and assumed a new and more impactful role approximately every two years, transitioning from the Medical Director of Hospital Quality to the eight-hospital health system's Clinical Director for Clinical Resource Management and Information Systems, to a hospital Vice President for Medical Affairs and Regional Chief Medical Officer, and culminating as the health system's Senior Vice President and Chief Quality Officer.

This final role exposed him to consultants and the process of leading a major health system turnaround while helping take out $110M of costs from the $1.8B budget to avoid bankruptcy and keep the doors open.

He reflected on feeling down one day due to the difficult decisions that were being made and recalls the lead consultant suggesting that he should not focus on the various difficult cuts that were required but rather appreciate that they were saving a health system that will continue to employ many thousands of people and will continue to care for the citizens of Detroit for the future. This reframing of solving these significant financial challenges helped improve his job satisfaction and provided greater clarity in helping create solutions for the health system.

During the seven years at Wayne State University and Detroit Medical Center, he simultaneously wanted to learn the academic side of the business of medicine where he completed the American College of Physician Executive's

Certified Physician Executive Program, the Henry Ford Health System's Managed Care College certificate, an MBA from the University of Michigan, and an MPH in Clinical Effectiveness from Harvard University.

Dr. Ransom describes this time as his "first career," where he built his professional foundation through both classroom and practical experiences as an active clinician, researcher, author, teacher, professor, and executive. He learned how to get things done through an outcome and multidisciplinary team-oriented, enthusiastic leadership approach.

He describes his "second career" when he left Detroit to become a faculty member and Director for the Program for Healthcare Improvement and Leadership Development at the University of Michigan in Ann Arbor. He was quickly promoted from associate to a tenured full professor with appointments at both the University of Michigan Medical School's Department of Obstetrics and Gynecology and School of Public Health's Department of Health Management and Policy. He authored scores of peer-reviewed manuscripts and medical textbooks, procured substantial NIH, NSF, and VA funding to support his research on topics related to health disparities, clinical effectiveness, and healthcare management.

He had a passion for building the evidence-base in the emerging areas of cost-effectiveness analysis and healthcare delivery research to learn how to lead better and improve healthcare organizations. It was during this time that he was elected to serve on the Board and then as President of the American College of Physician Executives. He found the opportunity to conduct health management research, care for patients, influence health policy, and help develop approaches to support physician executive careers across the country as important and exciting—until a recruiter called.

After seven years at the University of Michigan, a recruiter called Dr. Ransom about a position for an organization he had never heard of. The recruiter explained that they were looking for a President of a state-supported academic health science center/medical school and Vice Chancellor for Health Affairs for the university system and hoped to identify and recruit a leader who had three criteria: a board-certified physician who could be licensed to practice medicine in the State of Texas, an academic leader with a strong history of NIH and other extramural research funding that demonstrated a history of building academic and research programs, and a person who had experience leading a turnaround for a troubled clinical enterprise. The University of North Texas Health Science Center was in critical condition, needing a turnaround to improve its clinical quality, research funding, and financial position.

During his seven years in this position, the organization tripled the number of patient encounters from just over 200,000 to nearly 600,000; turned the financial deficit of the physician practice plan into a 9% sustainable operating margin; and improved external measures of success, such as advancing its *US News and World Report* rankings in primary care, rural medicine, geriatrics, and family medicine programs to all sit between 15th and 28th nationally.

During his tenure, he and his team also created several new schools and colleges such as Pharmacy, Physical Therapy, and a PhD in Public Health and expanded every existing college, including doubling the class size of the medical school to help achieve the goal of expanding the supply of much-needed healthcare providers for the State of Texas.

Upon his departure from the role, the academic health science center had a strong balance sheet with sustained clinical enterprise profitability, doubled its faculty size to 421 full-time and 851 adjuncts, expanded the staff to 1,400, and doubled the number of students to 1,949 housed in five colleges, including Medicine, Public Health, Health Professions, Biomedical Sciences, and Pharmacy.

In this phase of his career, Dr. Ransom also learned how to lead people who had positions and roles in which he had zero experience or expertise, such as the campus police department and facility construction. The leadership skills necessary to lead an entire organization are very different from leading areas of personal expertise. He reflects,

> Developing a results-oriented culture that inspires diverse leadership talent that are willing to share their sometimes contradictory insights to help make the right decision requires a lot more people skills and EQ than being the smartest one in the room.

After seven years, he started to "get the itch for another career change." He moved from the University of North Texas to McKinsey and Company, where he became a strategy consultant and leader of the Southern Region of their healthcare payer/provider practice. During his time there, he learned how to advise clients as well as lead and impact change as a consultant rather than as an executive.

After a few years, he moved to Navigant consulting for the opportunity to lead their entire strategy practice as well as academic medical center practice, and then to PwC|Strategy& to serve as a Partner in their health industry strategy practice until reaching the firm's required retirement age, and then to Partner in Oliver Wyman's Health and Life Sciences strategy practice.

Over the course of his strategy consulting career, he has advised clients in most major U.S. markets, Canada, Mexico, Saudi Arabia, Jordan, Qatar, United Kingdom, Germany, Chile, China, and Australia, working on every continent except Antarctica, engaging in deep strategic, operational, and transformational change engagements too improve healthcare organizations capacity and capability to better care for patients.

He has worked with payers, providers, pharmaceutical companies, healthcare start-ups, and governmental entities around the world, both large and small, including most of the top 10 ranked health systems, children's hospitals, and medical schools based on *US News and World Report*. One engagement included leading the strategy and design for the entire healthcare system for a Middle Eastern country. For now, he has no desire to retire, and continues his ongoing work in strategy and turnarounds during this "fourth career."

During these four careers, Dr. Ransom has published more than 150 articles and 11 books, including three ob-gyn textbooks and three healthcare management texts, and has co-edited five editions of the leading healthcare quality book, *The Healthcare Quality Book: Vision, Strategy and Tools*.

He delivered more than 4,000 babies and completed 10,000 surgeries while helping train hundreds of medical students, residents, and fellows. He has served in many national leadership roles, such as President of the American College of Physician Executives, and as an active board member on multiple not-for-profit boards.

In his spare time, he has helped start a free medical clinic in the Maasai region of Tanzania, climbed many mountains across the globe such as Rainier and Kilimanjaro, become a PADI-certified SCUBA instructor, and had the opportunity to experience hundreds of dives.

He has been married for 44 years to Elizabeth Ransom, MD, an otolaryngologist who has also served in several senior physician executive roles. They have raised three children.

Dr. Ransom defines his professional leadership journey as four separate careers, each about seven to nine years in duration: (1) as an early/middle career executive, clinician, and researcher at Wayne State University/Detroit Medical Center; (2) a senior faculty member, clinician, researcher, and institute leader at the University of Michigan Health System; (3) a chief executive officer for an academic health science center and medical school and vice chancellor for a university system; and (4) as a leading strategy consultant.

In total, his entire career has led to increasing ways to positively impact the health and welfare of individual patients and the broader population. In career one, he affected hundreds of lives as a clinician and middle manager; in career two, he affected tens of thousands of lives by figuring out better solutions to care for patients through research; in career three, he further expanded impact by leading a large clinical enterprise that cared for several hundred thousand patients annually and helped train thousands of future doctors, physician assistants, researchers, pharmacists, physical therapists and public health leaders that will collectively impact millions of lives; and in career four, he further broadened his impact by working with more than 150 healthcare organizations to better care for millions of people across the globe.

He believes physician leadership is crucial to driving major improvements in the healthcare delivery system and advancing the health and welfare of our population:

> If you look at the top 10 health system systems in *US News and World Report*, eight are led by physician chief executives, and that is not a coincidence. If you look at the next 50, physician leadership is disproportionately high. Physicians, especially those trained in management and armed with the necessary people skills, are uniquely positioned to understand their organization's core mission and help realize better care for individual patients as well as improve the health and welfare of the communities they serve. Great leaders have a passion for leading their organization from the perspective of what's best for the organization rather than their personal success, and they learn how to lead people even when they don't fully understand how to do their job. They are constantly learning.

CONCLUSION

These 11 physician leaders differ in many ways. They happen to be diverse with respect to gender, ethnicity, religion, sexual orientation, age, work-setting, medical degree, region, and leadership journey. But they all have a least two things in common: They are leaders I have personally known and learned from, and they are authentic leaders.

In this book, I have explored various theories of leadership and analyzed physician leadership within those contexts. An emerging leadership theory is authentic leadership, developed around three distinct qualities: self-awareness, self-inquiry, and self-realization. Authenticity in leadership is rooted in being true to one's own ideals of leadership and ethical values, building self-awareness by using life stories for self-reflection and self-awareness.

Authentic leaders who are aware of their core values are unlikely to stray from them. The ancient Greek maxim to "know thyself" is the essential element of authentic leadership.

I hope you find the book useful in your own leadership journey. We need physicians to lead.

REFERENCES

1. Kaplan AS, Abongwa A. U.S. Hospitals Can No Longer Afford the Burden of Administrative Waste. Healthcare Financial Management Association, Aug 20, 2020. www.hfma.org/topics/financial-sustainability/article/u-s-hospitals-can-no-longer-afford-the-burden-of-administrative-.html.

2. Kaplan A. The Risks, Rewards of Taking Organizations 'Where They Haven't Gone Before.' Modern Healthcare. February 9, 2021. www.modernhealthcare.com/opinion-editorial/risks-rewards-taking-organizations-where-they-havent-gone

3. Hafferty FW, Castellani B. The Increasing Complexities of Professionalism. *Acad Med.* 2010;85(2):288-301.

4. Bick D, Bick SL, Dimmock DP, et al. An Online Compendium of Treatable Genetic Disorders. Am J Med Genet C Semin Med Genet. 2021; 187(1):48-54.

www.ingramcontent.com/pod-product-compliance
Lightning Source LLC
Chambersburg PA
CBHW070713220326
41598CB00024BA/3129